[redacted]

FORTIER—BERNOVILLE

Therapeutics of the diseases of Liver and of Biliary ducts

Translated by
Dr. RAJKUMAR MUKERJI
M.A., L.H.M.S.

B. JAIN PUBLISHERS (P) LTD.
NEW DELHI-110055

Reprinted 1996

Price : Rs. 20.00

Published by :
B. Jain Publishers Pvt. Ltd.
1921, Street No. 10, Chuna Mandi
Paharganj, New Delhi - 110 055 (INDIA)

Printed at :
J. J. Offset Printers
Wazirpur, Delhi

ISBN 81-7021-254-5

BOOK CODE B-2052

To

Dilip

Dadu

PREFACE

I have included in this book the translations of the articles of **Dr. Fortier-Bernoville** published in five special issues of l' Homoeopathie modern entitled "*La therapeutique homoeo-athique des affections du foie et voies biliaires*", No. 3, 1938, & Nos. 5, 7, 9, 11 of 1938,

One point is to be noted in the articles included in this book. The followers of l' Homoeopathie modern are the adepts of the neo-hippocratic school. They do not ignore the importance of Homoeopathic treatment based on the symptoms presented by the patient, but the cause that has created hepatic insufficiency is of primary importance to them. The different types of insufficiencies of liver have each of them specific be-havior. This specificity we may call biological specificity. In a patholgical trouble of the liver the biological specificity shows that it is only necessary to diagnose the disease and the patient, but it is also necessary to valorise the biological specificities that are in play. This idea of biological specificity, seems in the case of hepatic insufficiency and in other troubles, to be very fecund and gives some important possibilities of compre-hension.

Once the biological specificity is know there remains to take into consideration the exterior factors : the past which has caused the insufficiency and the future which may cure it. Then there are different other factors : cosmic, meteorologic, hygienic, dietetic, microbian, social, psychological etc. When the doctor has well studied these factors he will find out the curative agent.

The second point that should be noted is about "Drainage and Canalisation". In these articles the reader will find some very clear examples of drainage. On this subject, I will ask my readers to consult my translation "what we must not do in Homoeopathy " in which a chapter on Drainage and canalisation is included, where the principle of drainage is fully described.

Complexism in homoeopathy is not new though it is looked down by the unicists. Most of the Homoeopaths of France in this regard follow the theory of drainag as expounded by **Dr. A. Nebel of Lausanne.** In one word we may say that the theory of drainage and canalization is nothing but to help our Polychrests or Ground remedies to act without causing aggravation because of their powarful eliminatory function. In this connection let me say that antidotes are helping remedies, they do not destroy the action of remedies which they antidote. The ahtidotes act like an "Umbrella" checking the powerful heat of the sun.

After the publication of may translation "What we must not do in Homoeopathy", I have received many letters from may Colleagues of India asking me to write in detail about drainage and canalisation. They will find in these articles some beautiful examples of drainage canalisation. The drainage of the abdomen described in a drawing will be specially interesting to them. When the 3rd ed. of the above book will be printed I will add some more details on the subject.

With these few words I leave the book to the readers for their own judgment. But I must say that in my practice I have found this method much more useful then the system of the unicists, which is sometime disheartening and dangereus as well.

CHANDANNAGAR.
Hooghly, W. B.

R. K. MUKERJI

CONTENTS

HEPATIC DYSFUNCTION: REMEDIES OF MORBID TEMPERAMENTS OF THE HEPATICS.

Multiple are the stages that are encompassed within the field of the word "Hepatic insufficiency".

1. First of all it is described by the name of "Hepatism" (de Glenard) an ensemble of troubles that helps to reveal a fragility of the liver acquired or very often hereditary, weakness that predisposes the individuals to liver affections in general and to many other diseases such as asthma, urticaria, migraine, uricemia, biliary lithiasis, rheumatism, neuralgias etc. The term "Hepatism" is replaced by some authors by the word "Arthritism". It has now been considered as a real diathesis. The process of palpation of the liver by the thumb (Glenard), periodic measurement of the height of the liver on the mammary line, the researches for the digestive troubles of reflex origin (aversion for fat, salivation, pain of the right shoulder), allow the use of the word "Hepatism", a very seducing clinical conception, but which is controversial at present. However we cannot deny the possibility of the fragility of the liver, as the first step towards the functional trouble of that gland.

2. Secondly, it was said and still it is said about the extraordinary frequency of cases labelled as Hepatic insufficiency. Habitually as regards thyroid, suprarenal or other glandular organs, one speaks about hyperfunctions and hypofunctions. As regards liver, there is only the insufficiency of the function which one can take into accunt clinically. But the functions of the liver is multiple and their classification differs with different authors. Every year something new is discovered. It is for this reason the word hepatic insufficieney is a vague term, very wide, which may be charac-

terised by some numerous different syndroms. It is this that was shown in the International Congress of hepatic insufficiency which was held last year in Vichy. It was right to have wanted to characterise the cases of insufficiency or hypofunction of liver, not only by current clinic, but some researches, some physiological tests, allowing a solid and quantitative basis of appreciation.

3. It is then perceived that the techniques proposed for characterising the hepatic insufficiency is only valuable in certain limited cases:

(a) The great insufficiency for grave type of jaundice, which differs, what is curious, from hepatectomy. Grave toxic hepatitis (*Phosphorus*, *Apiol*, *Cicophane* etc.) or ifectious, have augumentation of azotemia, of polypeptides, of amino acids and of residual nitrogen of the blood, and moreover some important haemorrhages, with delay in coagulation and the time of blood flowing increased.

(b) The great hepatic insufficiency as a consequence of hepatectomy characterized by hypo-glycemia, sudden fall of the glucose in blood, fall of the quantity of urea in the blood and urine, by augumentation of ammonia in the urine, amino acids, polypeptides of the blood and of the bilirubinemia.

(c) Hepatic insufficiency of organic diseases of the liver hepatitis by infections or intoxications, cirrhosis at the beginning). In these cases the treatment of the hepatic insufficiency is unstable and difficult to realize with elimination of all possible causes of error.

) Finally there are numerous cases of so-called hepatic insu iency which the Prof. Cheray calls "false medicomunc e". These are multiple observations that the profanes and ev the doctors believe to have related to hepatic insufficiency, they are very often really some intestinal statistics because hronic intestinal affections secondarily cause hepatobiliary re ns.

Some cases of chronic hepaitc congestion (great eaters, great drinkers, amibiasis) or chronic cholecystitis cause secondary hepatobiliary reactions which are so-called "insufficiency".

(4) In all these cases, the tests and the researches are negative. There is only the clinical picture(dirty tongue, bad smelling breath, bitter taste in the mouth, constipation alternating with diarrhoea, big liver, urobilinuria, hunger pain dermatoses, pruritis, chill, headache, asthenia, insomnia, postprandial somnolence etc.). Prof. Chiray shows with reason that in all these cases some rational treatments of the intestinal stasis, of typhocolitis, non-lithiasic cholecystitis, and other causes, cause rapid disappearence of the digestive and biliary symptoms. One re-establishes the permeability of colons with liquid paraffin or some mucilages, by washing of the intestines etc. and may often cure the patient.

Even in Homoeopathy *Nux Vomica*, *Aloe*, *Mercurius solubilis*, *Podophyllum*, *Berberis*, *Bryonia*, act with success in such cases, as well as *Opium*, *Graphitis*, *Alumina*, *Taraxacum* and the remedies of constipation.

In a word if it is necessary to distinguish on the one hand the cases, which are not relatively frequent, of hepatic insufficiency which can be revealed by the tests from the multiple cases of simple congestion of liver secondary to some troubles of the intestine or of the bile duct.

But it is necessary to know the therapeutics of these two kinds of diseases and one cannot deny that in the second case, even if there is no hepatic insufficiency in the real sense of the term the functions of the gland are often troubled by *Hepatic Overwork* more or less slightly or temporarily.

It is for this reason the word "Dysfunction" characterises better the ensemble of cases of functional troubles of the liver, either because of the real insufficiency, deep or slight, or because of certain functions of the hepatic cells, without any real insufficiency.

II. Classification and Value of Researches and Tests of Hepatic Dysfunction.

Numerous techniques have been suggested in different times in order to characterise the functional troubles of the liver and specially to put in evidence the insufficiency of the liver. In reality these methods are aften deffiicient and difficult to apply in current practice and even the results given by the tests are far from having an absolute value. A large number of functions of the liver will require numerous biological examinations if one wishes to be complete.

Moreover for each function there are many evperiments from which it is difficult to chose one.

1. **Biliary Function.** It is classical to say that one can put in evidence the troubles of biliary functions by the verification of urobiline in excess in the urine, but at present it is disputable and all the authors do not admit that urobiline is due to a cellular lesion of the hepatics ; it is rather due to the obstruction of the biliary duct.

Another test is proposed by Prof. Chiray who recently, with the collaboration of his two collaborators, *Milorde Molochewich* and *Marcel Kipler*, has tried to determine the importance of the hepatic cell by studying the variation of biliary salts in the bile sucked out directly by duodenal tubage.

2. **Protidic Function.** Intestinal diastasis have disintegrated the big molecules of proteins into albumen and in peptones, then into polypeptides and finally into amino acids. It is with these acids hepatic cells may reconstitute the albumen meant for the organism and for the surplus they disintegrate the nitrogenous matters that pass to the phase of disemination, then by the ammonia phase, in order to become urea one may note the hepatic function by searching in the urine or in the blood the quantity of nitrogenated residues which are not completely transformed into urea. Formerly Albert Robin measured the co-efficient of nitrogen by the formula : nitrogen of urea in the urine/total nitrogen of urea. Then he finds

out the co-efficient of nitrogen of *Maillard* and the co-efficient of acidosis of *Lanzenberg* modified by *Derrient* and by *Feissinger.*

Even one can find out the quantity of residual nitrogen in the blood, or even the polypeptides and the amino-acids in the blood. There are a considerable number of examinations proposed for the dosage of all the compounds of nitrogen in the blood.

In order to understand at the same time the functional importance of kidneys and of the liver of almost all the persons suffering from chronic diseases after 40 years of age, I always do systematically chemical examination regarding the quantity of residual nitrogen, uric acid, chlorides, cholesterin and lipides in the urine. It is above all interesting to note the relations that exist between urea and cholesterin, as well between cholesterin and lipide. This helps to understand the so numerous cases of toximia due to the slowness of the nutritive function and function of the excretions.

3. **The anti-anaphylactic function** may be compared with periodic functions, thanks to which the liver holds the incom pletely disintegrated proteic substances. Some classical examinations such as digestive hemolysis, examination of the milk, may put in evidence the troubles of that anti-anaphylactic function.

4. **Glycogenic and glycopexic function.** It helps the liver to transform the glucose into glucocin and to conserve it and to distribute later on according to the need of the organism. One can put in evidence the troubles of this function by different tests, such as provoked hyperglycemia and specially thanks to glycosuria, hinted at first by *Bauer*. This test has a great importance specially in the research of hepatic insufficiency in surgery.

5. **Anti-toxic function.** The liver fixes and nutralises the toxins in order to eliminate them in the form of soluble products passing through the kidneys. It is proposed to put in

evidence this function by the examination of glycoronuria provoked, or by the measure of the oxydation of urinary Sulphur. These examinations are difficult to realize in current practic.

6. To that anti-toxic function one may compare the **chromatogenic function** of the liver which consists in the elimination by the liver some colouring substances as for example phenol-tetrachloride, phtalein, carmin-indigo, azoburine, Bengal rose, phenolchloresulpho-nephtaleine.

7. The blood-function or function of the liver on the coagulaation of blood, is at present disputable. It is not yet know whether fibrinogen is due to hepatic cells.

Some authors distinguish even at present the martial function, formation of the reserves of iron in the liver, in order to distribute it for helping the red globules.

Many clinicians were struck in all the countries by the weaknesses of the experiments on which is based the diagnosis of the hepatic insufficiency (Cheray). However it is necessary to look for the cases of latent hepatics, if not, one may risk submitting the patients to surgical instrumentation which become mortal in cases of undetected hepatic insufficiency. It is for this reason it is necessary to treat before, after the intervention of surgery, the patients who have clear symptoms of hepatic insufficiency found out by different experiments specially by galactosuria.

We are now going to pass in review the important remedies of morbid temperaments of hepatic dysfunction.

3. Remedies of Morbid Temperaments of Hepatic Dysfunction. Let us first of all think about the function of the liver in the organism.

The gland is at the sametime purifier, fixer of toxins, and transformer of foods which it degrades to seperate from them the products which are to be excreted and those that will be necessary for the economy of the organism. It is therefore an organ of the first importance in the cycle run by the substances that the living organism borrows directly or indirectly from the mineral kingdom.

"The living matter is composed of carbon, hydrogen, oxygen, nitrogen, sulphur, phosphorus, to which are added chlorides, potassium, sodium, calcium, magnesium. iron and accessorily the silicum and fluoride (Lambling). The other minerals are less important, at least quantitatively.

The carbon is borrowed by the living matter under the form of carbonic acid, hydrogen in water state, nitrogen from ammonia state, sulphur in the state of sulphuric acid.

As a consequence of the different operations for reduction and synthesis, the living matter builds from the organic substances some complex organic matters, proteins, fat, hydrate of carbon, combined with some mineral substances (chloride, sodium phosphate, potassium, magnesium etc.) for obtaining the immediate principles constituting the tissues and the organs of the living matters. The simple substances will generally be the homoeopathic remedies of the first importance.

Thus we find the three principal minerals, which are the principal remedies of liver : *Sulphur*, *Natrum*, *sulphuricum* and *Phosphorus*. Besides there are three other remedies.

Lycopodium. A vegetable substance, containing Sulphur and even Natrum sulphuricum in sufficient quantity and also some Phosphorus.

Sepia, Lachesis. Animal products, they are very complex but they are less important than the 4 other remedies.

Ammonium carbonicum. The important remedy of uremia as well as *Phosphorus* to which it is related, is not a ground remedy because it is hardly prescribed in high dilution, but it is better to mention it here.

Now we will understand well the value of remedies of mineral origin for the treatment of troubles due to hepatic insufficiency. *Lycopodium*, which contains, *Sulphur*, *Natrum sulph*, and some *Phosphorus*, will be the remedy of the first importance in the hepatic insufficiency.

After these three minerals we may consider that the important remedies of morbid temperament in the dysfunction of the liver are the same as those that will be indicated in all the affections of the lesions of the hepatic cells. Let us mention here that there is not a difference in the degree of intensity of symptoms observed between functional troubles and impairment of the organ.

It is necessary to consider, in my opinion, 6 principal remedies of morbid temperament of the hepatics.

Three minerals : *Sulphur, Natrum sulphuricum, Phosphorus.*

One vegetable : *Lycopodium.*

Two animal products : *Lachesis* and *Sepia.*

Sulphur does not play in the treatment of the diseases of liver as important a part as that of **Lycopodium, Phosphorus, Natrum Sulphuricum**. However suits well to some troubles co-existing with an active and transitory congestion of liver, or with general arterial congestion. Arteria hypertension. By extension and localisation, hypertensions in the sphere of veins (portal), veins of the lower cava and of abdominal veins and its branches. This *General Abdominal Congestion* may be one of the symptoms of a tendency towards cancer with localisation in the abdomen. *Bleeding Hemorrhoids*, incessant or periodical bleeding, are clear symptoms of **Sulphur**. This flow of blood is a *Real Safety Valve* of a *Psoric State* or often plethoric.

The psora is often expressed by :

—**Periodic Cutaneous Eruptions,** eczema, *Urticaria*, furoncles and acne. All these eruptions are aggravated by washing.

—**Other Possible Phenomena of Eliminations** : epistaxis, periodic or continued, diarrhoea.

The sulphur organism should burn. It is the volcano. The mucous membranes are of red colour, specially of the orifices (lips, anus).

It has eruptions as a result of *Centrifugal Power* of this temperament, if the patient cannot drain himself in any other way.

The pains are of *Burning Type*, specially burning in the gastric region.

—Burning of the feet, *The Patient Searches For a Cool Place on the bed.* The sensation of combustion is such that the patient cannot fast, fasting is unbearable. *Goneness Feeling in the Stomach* towards 11 a.m. ; must eat at that time, which causes amelioration. No symptom of the liver. The liver is temporarily big and congested, diminishes soon by a high dillution, 200 or M (Korsakov).

The symptoms are general and digestive.

One important symptom *Of Proteopexic Troubles. The Milk is very Badly Tolerated.* Another symptom : cannot digest eggs (the yellow of the egg contain *Sulphur* and *Phosphorus*). Sometimes, sugar, farinaceous foods and starch are not tolerated. (Let us note that the milk and yellow of the egg are cholagogs)

Light cat's nap, wakes up by the least noise. Insomnia from 2 to 5 a.m.

If there is diarrhoea, aggr. at 5 a.m. ; the patient must make haste.

The stools may be colourless, diarrhoeic or not.

Painful tension in the region of liver. This symptom is rarely spontaneous, often it does not exist, caused only by pressure.

The complementaries and drainers of *Sulphur* will be :

Nux Vomica. For the intestines.

Aloe. For the rectum (It is choleretic), Dr. Nabel's ca nalizer of this organ.

Podophyllum. Choleretic for Charbol in ponderable dose. Elective action on the duodenum and secondarily on the rectum.

Megnesia sulphurica. Very powerful cholagog and choleretic in heavy doses.

Anacardium. When the sensation of empty feeling in the stomach is better by eating.

Mercurius has humid mouth with thirst, aggr. by the heat of the bed. Sweats do not ameliorate.

Has also close relation with *Lycopodium* (the vegetable Sulphur) and with *phosphorus* (troubles of the composition of blood).

Sepia. (Portal hypertension)

Natrum Sulphuricum. Hydrogenoid constitution. *Phosphorus* is distantly related to it.

Natrum Sulphuricum. suits specially to hydrogenoid patients.

Natrum Sulphuricum and ***Magnesia*** *carbonicum* are good choleretics (Charbol), therefore acting on the production of bile from the interstitial lymph and laminary system.

Aggr. during humid times and in humid places, in marshy lands and in unhealthy places. Better by humid heat (Ipecac). Retention of water by the liver and by the tissues (peri-visceral oedema). Gouty constitution (possibility of uricemia).

Hepatic Symptoms. Sensation of pressure on the region of liver.

—Pain caused by palpation.

—Fullness in the region of liver ; aggr. by the least pressure by a belt and by any tight thing on the body (Lachesis).

—A possible blood-symptom : diminution of the viscosity of blood.

—Chloride retention (blood, urine) but very frequently *Hyper-cholesterinemia* with a hydrogenoid state, needing water to saturate chloride.

—It acts on water metabolism. Troubles of thyroid and lymphophysery glands.

Tongue greenish-gray, salty taste of gastric and pharyngial mucous.

Voracious appetite, followed by regurgitations and loss of appetite. Nausea in the morning.

Flatulence. Thirst for very cold, icy drinks.

Borborygmus. Intestinal gas that one cannot expel.

Pressing diarrhoea, after break-fast, yellowish, with gas

Intestinal pains, aggr. while lying on the left side (Sepia). Tendency to warts

Natrum sulphuricum is therefore a very good remedy of the liver. It is telated to :

—*China.* Acts on the excess of cholesterinemia.

—*Cholesterinum.* Same (high dilutions)

—*Lecithin.* Antagonist of cholesterin. To be used in gross dose as a cholagog.

—*Podophyllum.* Choleretic ; morning diarrhoea, yellowish stool. Action on the duodenum and rectum.

—*Calcarea carbonica.* May act also in hydrogenoids or persons suffering from cholesterinemia.

—*Dulcamara.* Hydrogenoid constitution. Gout alternates with digestive symptoms.

Nux Vomica. A drainer of *Natrum sulphuricum.* Hydrogenoid for the intestines.

Kali carbonicum. Pricking pain in the liver as if from needles. Pain in kidneys. Weakness. Acts like Vichy water.

As a ground remedy *Natrum sulphuricum* is related to :

Sulphur. Congestion of liver.

Lycopodium. Has *Natrum sulphuricum* in its composition.

Phosphorus. Action on cholesterin.

Lachesis.

Sepia. May sometimes be hydrogenoid.

Like *Sulphur, Natrum sulphuricum* has a clear centrifugal action : elimination.

Action on the *biliary function.* It is to be noted that one of the biliary salts, *Taurocholate* contains at the sametime Sulphur and Sodium like *Natrum Sulphuricum*, which itself is choleretic, therefore acting by the formation of bile salts in the tissues.

Phosphorus. Very important remedy of the liver, not very well known by homoeopaths, because it is thought to be dangerous.

In fact, it is dangerous only in tuberculosis of the lungs and of the larynx. It is a remedy of degeneration of fat. (Kali bichromicum and phloridine). Therefore it suits less to ordinary insufficiency of the liver. It is rather a remedy of cirrhosis, deep, acute insufficiency of the liver (serious kinds of jaundice) or chronic affection (with cholecystitis).

Thirst for very cold water. Hungry immediately after meals. Sour taste and eructations after meals.

Gastric pains amel. by cold foods. Hiccough, sensation of emptyness in the stomach, great sensitiveness in the epigattrium.

Liver big and painful. Icterus. Colourless stool, grayish white stool.

Grave jaundice. Haemorrhages. *Retarded Menstruation. Diminution of Coagulability.*

Action on the blood-function of the liver (perhaps action on the formation of fibrinogens)

Purpura (no other action on the skin)

Sensation of emptyness and coldness in the abdomen.

Acts on the pancreas. Acute or chronic pancreatitis.

Sometimes constipation of hard, dry and narrow stools. Sometimes weakning diarrhoea, painless, mixed with small solid white particles. Acts on hepatic insufficiency of olds suffering from bile stone, or from cholecystitis, with chronic pancreatitis.

Action on uremia. Acts more on endocrinal liver than on exocrinal liver.

Action also on *Alcoholism* (*Sulphur*, *Lachesis*, *Lycopodium*, *Nux vomica*):

Action on bones; organic fat; walls of blood vessels, parenchymas, nerve cells.

Relations : As complementary, related to :

—*China*. Reenforces *Phosphorus*. Has action like *Phosphorus* on cholesterin.

—*Berberis*. Drains *Phosphorus* towards urines.

-*Ricinus Communis*. Excellent action on nausea.

—*Bryonia*. According to the modalities.

—*Digitalis*. Cardiac liver, and accordeon liver, with *China* and *Phosphorus*.

—*Chelidonium*. For cholesterinemia. Should be given in M or DM.

—*Lecithin*. In ponderable doses. Antagonist of cholesterin.

—*Lutein*. Cholecystitis and lithiases of women during menopause or during pregnency.

—*Arsenicum album.* Restlessness and prostration, better by heat.

—*Crotalus horridus.* Grave jaundice. A remedy of yellow fever.

—*Chloroforme.* In grave icterus.

—*Kali bichromicum.* In fatty degeneration.

—*Phlorizine.* In fatty degeneration.

As ground remedy compare with :

—*Lycopodium.* Insufficient, small liver. A remedy of "bitter" of the bile than of the "sugar".

—*Sulphur.* Very distant.

—*Natrum Sulphuricum.* Cholesterinemia.

—*Lachesis.* Simillar action on blood. General insufficiency. Forms cholesterin.

—*Sepia.* Distant relation. Portal hypertension.

Lycopodium. Classical insufficiency of the liver with more or less discrete phenomena of *Retention of Bile.* It is also a remedy of ground of familial cholemia of Gilbert (with *China*)

Hereditary Syphilitics, which creates some tenacious troubles of liver function, has the need for *Lycopodium* as much as *Luesinum*, *Aurum metallicum* and the salts of *Mercury*.

We have shown sometimes ago that *Lycopodium*, with *Sepia* were the ground remedies corresponding very often to the *Infantile Anorexia.* This affection, is sometimes called mental, really has some clear symptoms of hepatic insufficiency corresponding to the symptoms of this remedy.

Lycopodium is also a habitual remedy of hepatic insufficiency caused by alcoholism and of Laennec's *Atrophic Cirrhosis* : cirrhosis with sclerosis=*Lycopodium*; Cirrhosis with degeneration=*Phosphorus.*

It is now classic to compare the spores of *Lycopodium* with the anatomic representation of hepatic lobule. The similarity is striking.

Lycopodium is a moss of which the spores are inert, and considered with reason as such in Allopathy in gross doses, are capable of becoming, when diluted and dynamised, an extremely active remedy ; so active that it is dangerous to prescribe in high dilution even in the 30th, to patients having torpid liver (general insufficiency, cirrhosis, cholecystitis, acute or chronic grave jaundice). On the contrary in habitual cases of hepatic insufficiency, *Lycopodium* is the best remedy.

In fact *Lycopodium* seems to be a remedy *par excellence* for overworked liver. It is for this reason it is a remedy of the "bilious" type to whom corresponds its mental characteristics.

Mentally : apprehension, weakness of memory, forgets words and syllables while writing. Very irritable. Becomes easily angry. Frequent underlining of phrases, in letters that the writes.

Likes to write in violent terms or even in obscene terms, if they are expressive.

Sad in the morning while waking up (contrary, *Sulphur*). Jaundice after anger (*Colocynth, Chamomilla*). The liver is the gland of anger.

Digestive Tract. Dry mouth without thirst. Weak digestion. Incomplete burning eructations rising up to the pharynx.

Prefers hot food and drink (*Cyelidonium* and *Arsenic* ; contrary *Phosphorus* and often *Sulphur*). Gastric and intestinal distension. Retention or emission of abundant intestinal gas.

Constipation of insufficient stools. *Painful Hemorrhoids.*

The action of *Lycopodium* in constipation is very mysterious.

Very often in the lower dilutions (3, 6, 12), *Lycopodium* ameliorates constipation (when it is indicated to *Lycopodium*).

Very often, in high dilutions or in medium dilutions (30, 200, M) *Lycopodium* aggr. the constipation (when it is indicated by the symptoms)

The phenomena exists also in *China*, *Chelidonium*, *Myrica*, *Nux vomica* etc...

What is the cause ?

Here is how we can interprete it.

The lower dilution of *Lycopodium* will act as a cholagog, and will eliminate the bile in the intestine more actively. Bile which slows down the heart in the cases of jaundice, on the contrary *Increases the Rapidity* of the intestinal transit, whence amelioration of constipation, but possibly also diminution of assimilation.

Inversely the intestinal transit would be slowed down, but with augumentation of the power of assimilation, in the case of hepatic insufficiency, ameliorated by *Lycopodium* in high dilutions. Whence the possible antagonism between the speed of elimination of bile and the power of assimilation, function of the liver cells.

Constipation in a person who has bad assimilation which is perhaps a defence reaction. Perhaps, the liver, by the help of bile, itself regulates the speed of transit exactly necessary to the necessity of assimilation ? It requires study.

Besides, we often see the bile extract, capable to overwork the liver and to cause some hepatic troubles either because of overwork or because of the insufficiency, perhaps because by activating the intenstinal transit ; intestines can no more bring back to the liver the biliary salt for recuperation (according to some authors)

Appetite of Lycopodium. Soon satisfied ; by a mouthful only. Dyspnoea caused by cabbage, greasy and farinaceous foods. Aversion to bread. *Desire for sugar* (*Argentum nitricum*, action on the glycogenic function *canno tolorate shellfish*).

Liver. Sensitive and painful, small often *hard* (Big liver Digitalis, *China, Phosphorus, Kali carbonicum* etc...). Hepatic pain *Aggravated by touch* ; while breathing, painful and heavy sensation on the liver. Point of Weihe, or painful point of *Lycopodium* is between the 2nd right or left intercostal space, at a distance of 2 cm from the border of sternum.

Yellow patches of the skin on the liver region.

Urine. Brick red sediment. Sometimes excess of uric acid, diminished or precipitated. *Lycopodium* will act on gouty diathesis like *Natrum sulphuricum* and *Lithium carbonicum.*

May go towards uremia, like *Ammonium carbonicum, Carbo veg., Arsenicum album, Phosphorus.* A good sign of *Lycopodium* : Urobilinuria. Has action also on acetonemy and acetonuria (Senna).

Circulation. Tendency to anervism, specially aortic.

Venous circulation. Naevi.

Erectile tumours.

One foot cold, the other hot.

Sleep. Cannot sleep on the right side (contrary *Sepia*)

General aggravation from 4 to 8 p.m. (from 4 to 5 a.m the urea in the urine increases.

Very marked *Rightsidedness.*

Relation of *Lycopodium* with.

Chelidonium. Very much similar. Bitter taste in the mouth. Pain in the scapulo-vertebral angle (right), into the point of scapula.

Myrica. Resembles to *Chelidonium.*

Chenopodium. Anthelmintic action on the labyrinth, deafness. Scapulo-vertebral pain like *Chelidonium.* Vertigo.

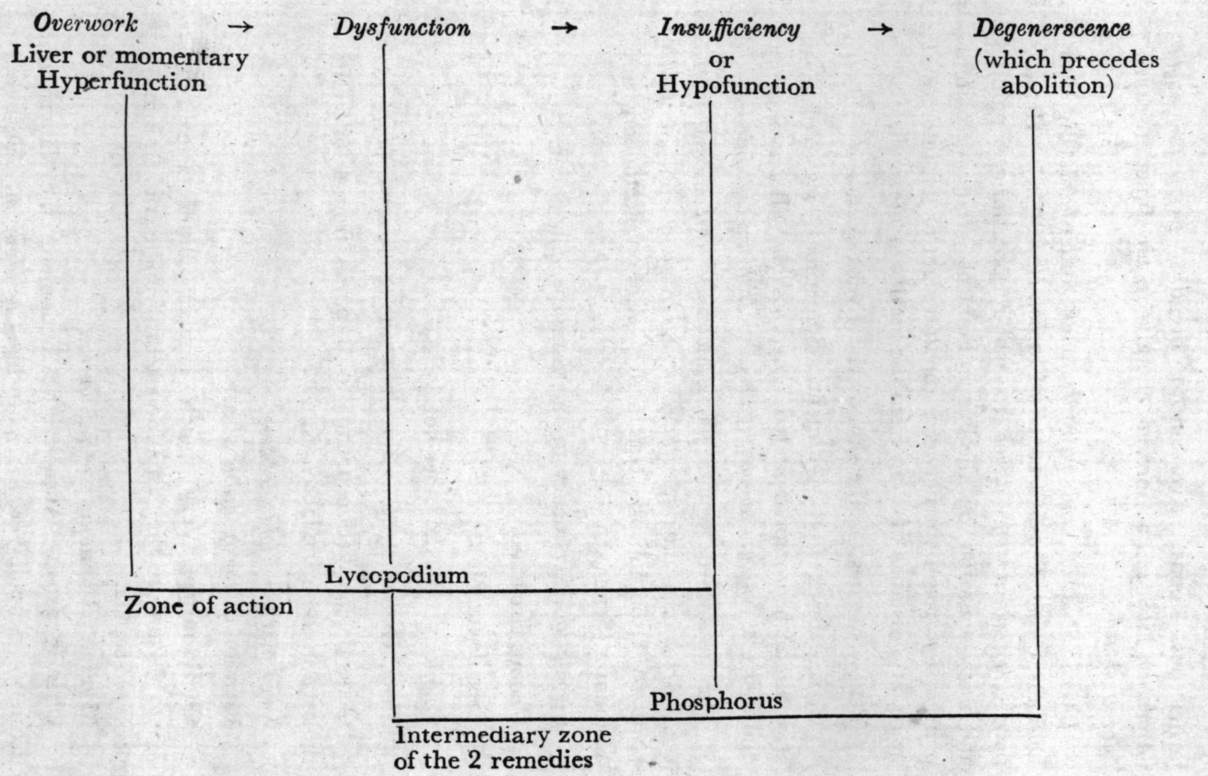
Overwork →
Liver or momentary Hyperfunction
Dysfunction →
Insufficiency or Hypofunction →
Degenerscence (which precedes abolition)
Lycopodium
Zone of action
Phosphorus
Intermediary zone of the 2 remedies

Chionathus. In jaundice

Mercurius solubilis, *Mercurius dulcis*, more or less disputable cholagogs.

China. It is antidote and complementary. Distention of the abdomen, generalised meteorism of the whole abdomen. Big liver, big spleen.

Arsenicum album. Complementary of *Lycopodium* and of *Phosphorus*.

Bryonia. According to the modalities. Better lying down on the painful side. Aggravation by respiration, like *Lycopodium.*

If aggr. caused by *Lycopodium* think of *China* (meteorism), or *Colocynthis* (pain after anger).

With ground remedies.

Sulphur and *Natrum sulphuricum*, very slight on the liver

Phosphorus. Deeper action (rather rightsidedness)

Sepia is between *Sulphur* and *Lycopodium*. *Lachesis* between *Phosphorus* and *Lycopodium* (*Lachesis*, leftsidedness)

The following schema may show the general action of *Lycopodium* and *Phosphorus* compared.

In schematising, let us say that *Lycopodium* acts on the whole field of hepatic lobule, probably on the protoplasma of hepatic cells and bile duct.

Phosphorus has for its field of action on hepatic cell, specially its nucleus (abundance of phosphorus in the nucleus).

Lycopodium should be drained through bile ducts.

Phosphorus should be drained specially through the central vein of the hepatic lobule and thence through the kidney.

There is no haemorrhage in *Lycopodium* while there is haemorrhage in *Phosphorus*, *Lachesis* and even in *Sulphur*.

Sepia has for its field of action the portal vein.

Sulphur on portal vein and on the whole arterial and venous system of the abdomen in general.

Natrum sulphuricum on blood serum and interstitial plasma of the tissues.

The last three remedies are only indirectly hepatics. Let us now define the field of action of *Lachesis* which is very difficult.

Lachesis. Less important in liver diseases than *Lycopodium* and *Phosphorus.* But it is necessary to think of it in cases of insufficient liver.

It is a remedy of Correlations, the function between the Liver and the Blood.

It is a remedy of Correlations of the function between the Liver and Sympathetic Nervous System.

Mentality. Logorrhoea, loquacity. Excitation, then depression (like Phosphorus). Suspicious, jealous, vindictive. Mania. Macabre dreams, dreams of death. The liver is the gland of jealousy. *Lachesis* is also a remedy of jealousy (sexual), of envy. Step-mother type, jealous of the step-daughter.

(Other remedy of jealousy, Hyocyamus). Menopause. Remedy of overwork (mental), mental shocks (efforts of creation, invention, berevement sorrow).

General Aggr. during Sleep. The sympathetic nervous system is never at rest. When the parasympathetic predominantes: suffocation while sleeping. Aggr. in the morning after waking up.

Vertigo. Gushes of heat. Headache (vertex), aggr. by sun.

Lips are purple or blue, livid.

Desire for oysters and alcohol.

A remedy of alcoholism (*Sulphur, Phosphorus Lycopodium, Gelsemium, Nux vomica*).

Lachesis rather Characterises the overwork of Nerves and Sympathetic system with Glandular overwork.

Liver Sensitive. Cannot keep anything tight around the body (Natrum sulph.), around the *Neck* or around the *Chest.* Abdominal tympanism, should loosen the clothes.

Constipation of foetid stools.

Haemorrnoids (*Phosphorus*) of decomposed blood.

Purple haemorrhoids, with constrictive pains.

General amel. during menses.

Hepatic troubles during menopause (*Lutein, phosphorus, Cholesterinum*)

Possible purpura.

In summary, in *Lachesis*, action on the blood ; unbalanced humours. Related to *Phosphorus* by its action on blood ; to *Lycopodium*, which comes before and after it by its action on the liver ; to *Sulphur* in arterial hypertension of women during menopause ; to *Sepia* by its action on the two poles : Liver-Organs of the lower abdomen.

Other relations :

Arsenicum Album. Restlessness and prostration.

Muriatic acid. Haemorrhoids.

Digitalis. Slow pulse, trigeminal pulse. Arythmia.

China. Very weakning haemorrhage of long duration.

Arnica. Traumatisms.

Ignatia Paradoxal symptoms. Sympathetic dislocation.

Vipera. Important action on the liver. Compare with *Ricinus* : big liver, as if it is going to burst. Cardiac oedema. Like *Lachesis* action on the veins. *Menopause.*

Sepia. A remedy-type of *portal hypertension.*

Sulphur, Lycopodium specially, sometimes *Natrum sulphuricum* and *Lachesis* have also portal hypertension of lesser degree.

What is the characteristic of *Sepia*? *Atony,* like all other medicines of *Generalised Venous Insufficiency* (Pulsatilla), or localised (Sepia). The last two remedies act every time when the organism intensely undergoes the law of heaviness.

Pulsatilla. suffers from this law everywhere, specially in the extremities : hands, feet, legs.

Sepia in the abdomen and in the lower abdomen, from the liver to the uterus and to rectum, whence its action on the liver, on the belly, on the anus, uterus and vagina.

The liver is big, painful, heavy ; aggr. of pains and uneasyness lying on the left side, sensation as if the liver is going to fall down from the right to the left under the influence of the heavyness. Tendency to *Prolapsus of the Anus, Sensation of a Ball in the Anus.* Constipation, stools are hard and large, or small balls, oozing and sometimes bleeding haemorrhoids.

Belly, *Swollen, Distended, Painful, Relaxed, Hanging.*

Requires a belt. Multiple ptosis.

Sensation of uterine "bearing down", or falling of the uterus.

Sometimes real prolapsus of the uterus.

Relaxed sphinister ani. Troubles of menstruation, irregular delayed or rare, early or profuse. Vagina, painful during coitious.

Weakness of the back. Pain in the back during menses.

In men *Congestion of Prostrate.*

General weakness. *Troubles of Suprarenal Gland, Hypoactivity.*

Skin. Yellow patches on the face (rings around eyes, horse shoe rings around cheeks and around the mouth. Patches on the abdomen, big dark patches (if small *Lycopodium*). Herpes. Eczema.

Mentality full of darkness sad, melancholic, sees none. Indifferent. Recoils within herself. Wishes to remain alone. Indolence, indifferent to others, anxious for her own self. Apathetic, but not wicked ; everything irritates her ; everything annoys her. No anger.

Vertigo. Headache. Tongue white. *Sensation of Emptyness in the Stomach not better by eating.*

Aggr. 11 'o'clock in the morning and at 6 in the evening or (4 to 6).

Amel. after sleep (contrary Lachesis)

Perversion of Taste. Foods taste salty, salty taste in the mouth. Desires for vinaigre and condiments.

Aggr. by milk, boiled milk.

Nausea and vomitting. Dirty tongue, posterior half.

Relation of Sepia.

Nux vomica. Intensifies action of *Sepia.* Portal congestion like *Sulphur* and *Sepia* (place between the two)

Nux moschata.

Gelsemium.

Helonias.

Aloe.

Pulsatilla, the antidote.

Berberis.

Lilium tigrinum.

Murex purpurea.

Is related to :

Sulphur. Portal hypertension.

Natrum sulphuricum. When she is hydrogenoid. Also to *Thuja.*

Lachesis for genital troubles.

Lycopodium. Antidote, antagonism with *Sepia.* But they proceed from one to the other.

Phosphorus. Phosphorus is a remedy of prolapsus. *Sepia* for the relaxed condition. *Phosphorus* for degeneration.

Such are the 6 remedies of the ground of hepatic dysfunction and of the organic defects of the liver.

Let us now see what are the remedies that seem to correspond to each of the principal troubled functions of the liver.

Whatever may be the remedies indicated for the liver let us recall here the rule :

In lower dilutions, the action is centrifugal ; in high dilutions the action is centrifugal and centripetal at the sametime.

In lower dilutions, action on the liver as an organ of excretion.

In high dilutions, action on the liver as an organ of secretion, an endocrine.

This rule is particularly true for substances used as cholagog and choleretic.

1. Troubles of Biliary Function. LYCOPODIUM, *China, Sulphur, Natrum sulphuricum* and *Phosphorus.*

And *China, Digitalis, Myrica, Berberis, Chelidonium, Mercurius dulcis, Podophyllum, Chionathus, Magnesia sulphurica.*

All these remedies may have jaundice as a symptom (except Phosphorus)

In cholesterinemia, the group of remedies is : *China, Phosphorus, Cholesterinum, Calcarea carbonica, Natrum sulphuricum, Graphitis.*

Elimination of cholesterol by the menstrual blood. (*Lutein, Lachesis* should correspond to Cholesterinum).

In retention of biliary salts : *Lycopodium, China, Chelidonium*

China. Everything tastes bitter even water. Liver is very often big. Big spleen. Loss of organic fluids. Anemia. Dehydration. Possible jaundice. Old malaria. China is antidote and complementary of *Lycopodium* after aggravation by the latter, in the form of meteorism. Generalised distension of the abdomen.

Digitalis. Cardiac liver. Weakness of the heart, specially of the right heart. Big congested liver. Often icterus & cardiac arythmia.

Berberis. Left kidney painful to pressure. Troubled urine, red-brick sediment.

Chelidonium. Jaundice. Bitter taste in the mouth. Wants to eat and drink hot. Pain in the lower angle of the right shoulder blade.

Mercurius dulcis or solubilis. Painful big liver. Humid mouth. Tongue with imprint of teeth on the borders.

Chionathus, Myrica. Jaundice, colourless stools, related to *Chelidonium*.

Magnesia Sulphurica. In ponderable dose or in very small dose or in lower triturations an excellent cholagog or cholereic.

For biliary retention : *Chamomilla, Colocynthis*, remedies of acute liver pain, angry and irritable temperament like *Lycopodium*.

2. Glycogenic Trobules. It is difficult to fight these troubles with homoeopathic remedies having certain indication in this sense.

Lycopodium and Phosphorus will act here. Also *Iris versicolor, Lactic acid, Insulin, Glycerin, Sizyzium*. But the pancreatic troubles domintate if there is diabetis. The pathogenesis is less known.

Lycopodium will act here in medium or high dilutions while for the biliary troubles, it will act in lower dilutions.

In biliary function of elemiiation the cycle is as follows :

Here opposition of "bitter" function	muscles→hepatic artery→hepatic cells→ biliary ducts, bile. bile salts Intestine Give *Lycopodium*, 6, 12 (Korsakov)

In centripetal glycogenic function the cycle will end thus.

And of the "sugar" function	Intestine→portal veine→hepatic cells→ lobular veins→veins→muscles (glycogenic function)→upperliver→kidney (uropoietic function) Give *Lycopodium*, 30, 200, M.

To the troubles of the elaboration of nitrogen seems to correspond : *Phosphorus* as well as *Lycopodium, China, Ammon carb.* and possibly also *Urea, Uric acid* (to try)

Moreover *Berberis, Baryata muriatica, Solidago* etc.—for drainage.

We will find these remedies again in the repertory on the elimination of excess of urates or precipitates.

If there is acetonemia : *Senna, Belladonna, Lycopodium, Calcarea muriatica, Causticum.*

4. For the function of antitoxic troubles : *Arsenicum album,* should often be indicated; alimentary intoxications when there are its indications. Restlessness, prostration; aggr. at 1 'o' clock at night and from midnight to 3 a.m., periodicity, diarrhoeic stools, blackish and small, cadaveric smell, intoxication by spoiled foods.

In other cases : *Phosphorus, Lycopodium, China, Antimonium crudum, Zanziber, Veratrum album, Colocynthis.*

Nux vomica. Sedentarism. Desire for stimulation, which does not only ameliorate momentarily but also as a consequence the patient feels worse.

For anti-anaphylactic function, it is very difficult to find sure remedies. To be studied in the **Materia Medica.** All sorts of remedies may be indicated. Specially *Arsenicum album* and *Thuja.*

Finally troubles of blood-function. We may use *Phosphorus* and *Lachesis.*

Both have hemorrhages (*Lycopodium* has not; *Sulphur* and *Sepia* have because of portal hypertension; *Sulphur*, bleeding ulcers, a safety valve for psoric diathesis).

Phosphorus. Possible grave jaundice. Slow coagulation of blood.

Purpura.

Thirst for very cold water. Sensation of goneness in the stomach.

Acute and deep hepatic insufficiency—grave or chronic icterus—chronic cholecystitis.

China, the complementary with *Ricinus communis Bryonia*, *Berberis* etc.

Lachesis. Aggr. after sleep, amel. during menses and by all kinds of blood discharge.

Logorrhoea, loquacity, jealousy, mistrust.

Dream of death.

Cannot bear anything tight on the body, around the neck, and around chest.

Such are the remedies which we can think of for the different troubles of hepatic functions.

But it is very difficult in the present development of biological and chemical sciences to fight these different functions and troubles, by remedies because we want in homoeopathy complete experimental works on the question.

Therefore let us stick to our **Materia Medica** which we should study deeply. The indications that I have just mentioned are my personal opinions, having only explicatory value. The future will prove them.

HOMOEOPATHIC PRACTICE OF DRAINAGE IN THE TREATMENT OF LIVER DISEASES AND THE DISEASES OF THE BILE DUCT

The most important natural outlets for elimination or for drainage are three : The digestive tract, urinary tract and the skin.

The urinary tract is the most important of all. It is at the sametime qualitative and quantitative. Sometimes one can live for a longtime without passing stools but one cannot live even eight days without passing urine.

The digestive tract, specially rectal is also very important quantitatively. In therapeutic it is much more easy to open the digestive barrier than the reno-vesical barrier It is partly a question of the surface, the wide surface of the intestinal epithalium, mucous of the small intestines and of colons.

The cutaneous outlet serves to eliminate periodically than continually : sweats, sebum, heat, eruptions. It is at the sametime an outlet for surface elimination, but rather qualitative, and before all depending on the movements of the individual or on the exposition to the sun and to cold and air. It also depends on the conditions of the surounding.

It is necessary to study the function of the liver as well as the drainage by the help of all these three tracts : digestive urinary, cutaneous.

On the other hand the different homoeopathic remedies will be indicated according to the meaning of drainage of which the liver, the laboratory of the organism, the biggest organic gland, is the point of departure.

Thus as for example *Phosphorus* and its satellites will be used for the elimination through : Liver→Circulatory tract→ Kidney.

On the contrary *Sulphur* and its complementaries act better in the passage : Liver→Billiary tract→intestines.

Abdomen, Drainage And Canalisation—

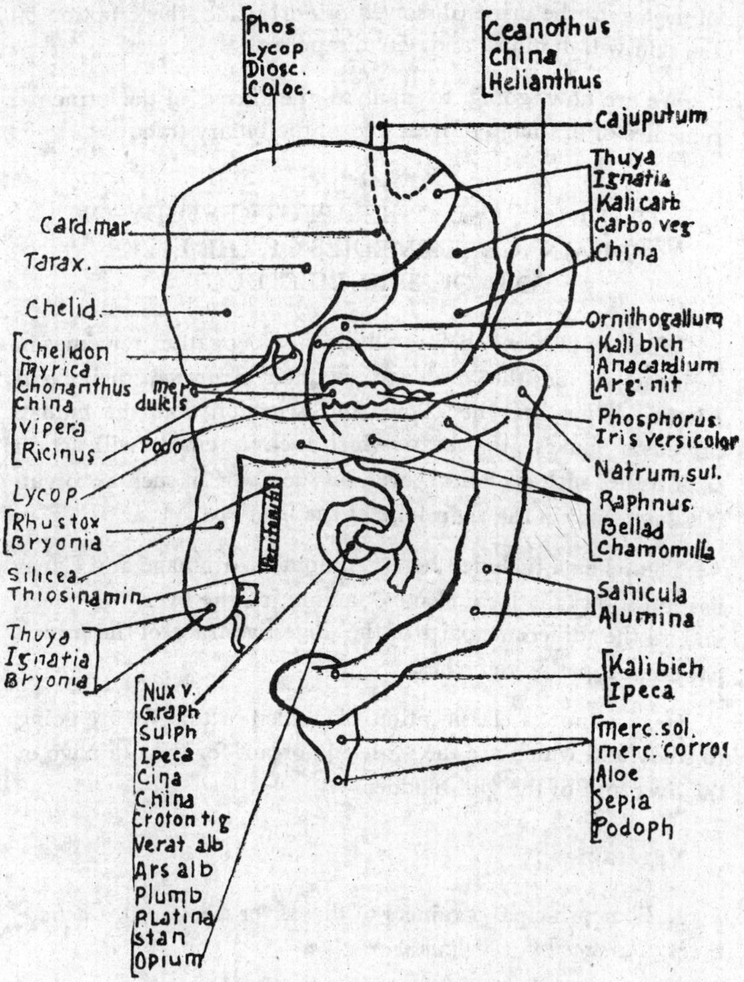

Other examples : Berberis 3 or 6 acts on the hepatic cells, on the kidney and on the skin. If this remedy is used in hepato-renal troubles, the kidney is helped causing an increase of elimination through the skin (by pruritis or by the reappearence of an old eczema). On the contrary the drainage, derivation of Nebel : *Fumaria* plus *Saponaria* lx controls the skin and seems to eliminate through the urinary tract. Similarly in urticarea, *Urtica urens* 6 will cause an elimination of urates in the urine (dissolved or not) while the eruption on the skin will diminish and will disappear.

We are now going to analyse the effects of the principal remedies of drainage of liver and of the biliary tract.

CLINICAL AND THERAPEUTIC STUDY OF DRAINAGE : REMEDIES OF THE LIVER AND OF THE BILE DUCT

What conditions before all the homoeopathic remedies in their action on the drainage, is their *Tropism*, their *Local Elective Action* and the choice and selection that the human organism makes, thanks to which such a remedy will act on such tissue, such region or even on such part of such an organ (*Chelidoinum* on the right lobe of the liver etc....)

The schema included here : Abdomen, drainage and Canalisation shows the local elective action, on the liver, the spleen and on the different parts of the digestive tract of the principal homoeopathic remedies.

Here is now a classification of remedies that we are going to study and which are the most important for the drainage of the liver and of the gall-bludder.

Vegetables :

1. Four principal drainers of the Liver : *Solidago*, *Chelidonium*, *Taraxacum*, *Carduus marianus*.

2. Six drainers of bile ducts and of the liver : *Hydrastis Chionathus*, *China*, *Myrica*, *Berberies*.

3. Four remedies of painful spasms of the bile ducts. *Colocynthis, Dioscoria villosa, Bryonia, Chamomilla.*

4. Four remedies of portal hypertension and of haemorrhoids in relation to liver troubles : *Podophyllum, Aloe, Aesculus hippocastum, Collinsonia.*

5. Four other remedies of hepato-biliary troubles : *Ptelia Leptandra, Jugulans cinerea, Yucca filamentosa.*

6. Minerals : Eight mineral compounds : *Natrum phos., Natrum sulphuricum, Magnesia muriatica, Magnesia sulphuricum, Kali bichromicum, Kali carbonicum, Mercurius solubilis* and *Mercrius dulcis.*

And finally :

7. Two remedies which are to be placed separately for their particular action on cholecystitis, one vegetable and the other from the animal kingdom : *Ricinus communis* and *Vipera.*

Biochemic remedies :

Some organic substances such as *Liver extract, Bile extract, Biliary salts, Calculus biliaris, Cholesterinum, Lecithin, Lutein,* and the choleretics and cholagogs described by Charbol, *Polypode, Cynara scolymus, Combratum, Boldo,* and *Rosemary* etc.

Finally there exist numerous remedies of *Derivation* which act not only on the liver but also on the other organs.

Iric versicolor (Pancreas and intracephalic circulation).

Digitalis (heart and kidneys).

Dulcamara (locomotor system and conjunctive tissues)

Nux vomica. Canaliser of *Sulphur* on the small intestines (Nebel)

Antimonium crudum. Action on the intestines.

Arsenicum album. Universal action. Every age, all the tissues of all organs.

Ceonathus. Principal sphere of action on the spleen.

Sepia. Portal veins and lower abdomen.

Pulsatilla. General venous congestion and troubles due to incomplete digestion of facts.

Cyclamen. For the digestion of fact.

Solidago, Chelidonium, Taraxacum, Carduus Marianus.

Solidago. An important remedy of drainage, indicated tous by Burnett, and we of the French school use it specially; foreign homoeopaths, usé it much less. Even we use it as a routine, prescribing it whenever our therapeutic ideas are somewhat vague.

Solidago, though very interesting to use and is of the first importance among the remedies for the drainage of the outlets, is not however the only one and should not occupy an exaggerated place. It is a plant, which grows in the forest and dry grounds. It is not consumed as food, but however one can ingest it in a small quantity without any danger and the cattles often eat them. It blooms in August and in September.

Empirically it is used as a diuretic and you will find in the book on phytotherapy of *Leclerc*, a small chapter on it, which is interesting to read, but this does not teach us, Homoeopaths, anything, because the Phytotherapaths know much less than us about the plant. *Leclerc* has however indicated to us that a decoction of *Solidágo*, may give good results in enteralgia, diarrhoea, dysenteric stools with tenasmus and in infantile enteritis during dentition.

It is a remedy that acts by opening the *Renal Barrage* and secondarily the digestive barrage. It has a very mild action on the liver and also on the lower limbs and on the blood.

The reputation of *Solidago* comes from the fact that it checks the medicinal aggravation caused bv *Sulphur, Nux Vomica, Lycopodium.* It may be related to all the important ground remedies and even to all the medicines of the **Materia Medica.** It has no incompatibility. Every time you use it for opening the renal barrage and at the same-time you prescribe other remedies, ground remedies and functional remedies, you need not be afraid of incompatibility you may be sure that it will not hinder the action of other remedies. But you must know how to apply it. If you use it in very low dilution, 1x or 3x, you risk an irritation of kidney. If you use it in very high dilution, you will not open the renal barrage. On my part, after number of trials, I have settled on 3x, 5 drops every day before meal at noon. The decoction acts very mildly as diuretic and does not cause dysuria. You may give safely to some persons, a cup of the decoction in the morning. By doing so you will have a very mild action on the kidney and on the liver.

Some homoeopaths with Chiron, have the habit of not giving a high dilution but begins to prescribe at first some remedies of drainage for eight days before giving the high dilution.

Sometimes *Solidago* will allow you to have a digestive elimination, *i. e.* it will act mildly on the constipation. But this is not always the case. Sometimes *Solidago* does not at all act on constipation when on the contrary the urine increases generally. The color of the urine may change. After the prescription of *Solidago* the deposit in the morning may be abundant.

But this remedy may not be always enough for drainage of digestive apparatus and kidney and you are sometimes obliged to give a functional remedy which will act as a link between the ground remedies and the drainage remedies. This is specially true for *Lycopodium.* You know that this consti-

t d l b d—3

tutional or ground remedy causes often some aggravations specially in adults. In children you may prescribe it without any fear of danger. To an adult it is very often "shocking". The aggravation is rarely dangerous but sometimes annoying; it is either hypersthenic, or hyposthenic; it may cause spasms like that of *Colocynthis* or an abdominal distension like that of *China.* If your *Lycopodium* subject defends violently, if he is nervous having many mental symptoms of the remedy, an angry person, he may very well, after having the dose of *Lycopodium,* have on the next day some very violent spasmodic pains in the abdomen, specially with a spasm of transverse colon, and of small intestines; the pain is so violent that the patient is obliged to bend double. In this case, you will give also *Colocynthis* 6 or 30, repeated every hour or every two hours, at the same time as complementary and antidote of *Lycopodium,* as complementary it follows *Lycopodium,* as antidote it checks its bad effects.

In order to save your patient from aggravation, you may give one dose of *Lycopodium* 200 followed by *Colocynthis* 30, one granule every day. You can prescribe it preferably at 4 to 5 p.m., *i.e.* to say towards the time of the aggravation of *Lycopodium.*

Other patients may have distension of the abdomen from the next day, a real general acrocholia, tiresome and painful, generalised meteorism in the whole abdomen. There is a kind of very intense blockage. *China,* then antidotes the bad effects of *Lycopodium* and is also a complementary to it.

And if you are afraid that your patient may have both types of aggravation you are quite right to follow your high dilution by *Colocynthis* 30 and *China* 30 alternately. *Solidago* will drain *Lycopodium* and will be prescribed everyday at noon. This is a very simple formula of drainage in Homoeopathy.

We must recall here that what is remarkable in homoeopathic medicine is that even the homoeopaths who have long experience, do not know how a patient is going to react the fiirst time when it has been prescribed to him. You may take the entire responsibility of cure in future, but you can never say to a patient who comes to you for the first time : "This first treatment is going to cure you or cause amelioration". You know nothing. It is impossible to know how a patient will react. One knows it only during the second consultation. There is always an unknown one, only temporarily. This unknown one shows us the necessity of individualising each case and not to give ever a patient a prescription of confection instead of giving him the measured remedy.

There is no doubt that *Solidago* has the benefit of that reputation to check medicinal aggravation but we must not exaggerate its use and should not use it as a routine. As we have said just now, it opens the renal barrage. The patient micturates better, the eliminations are sometimes more concentrated but very often abundan. Sometimes however after *Solidago*, the quantity of urine does not increase, but the patient goes well. In the symptoms indicated by **Dr. Renard**, I believe, it should be insisted when you wish to give *Solidago* on the symptom of "feeling weak". The patient, from sometime, feels that he is becoming weak, he is losing his energy in work and his kidneys are sensitive to pressure.

Solidago has a Weihe point situated on the region of right kidney, on the surface of the triangle of Jean-Louis Petit. Sometimes the constipation auguments after having taken the medicine specially when the liver is insufficient. One should not be anxious for this, because it seems that constipation at the beginning of a treatment gives for sometime rest to the hepatic cells. There is produced a slowness of the intestinal transit; a diminution of bile secretion, but the overworked liver takes rest, the patient then goes better. Even when the patient goes no more to pass stools and some mechanical means become necessary, he will remaine good because his liver will be slow acting. This is a point on which we have much insisted. There is but one remedy with centrifugal action on the digestive sphere in all the dilutions. It is *Taraxacum*. *Lycopodium* is centrifugal only in 6 or12.

Now we come to the study of *Chelidonium*, *Taraxacum and Carduu Marianus*.

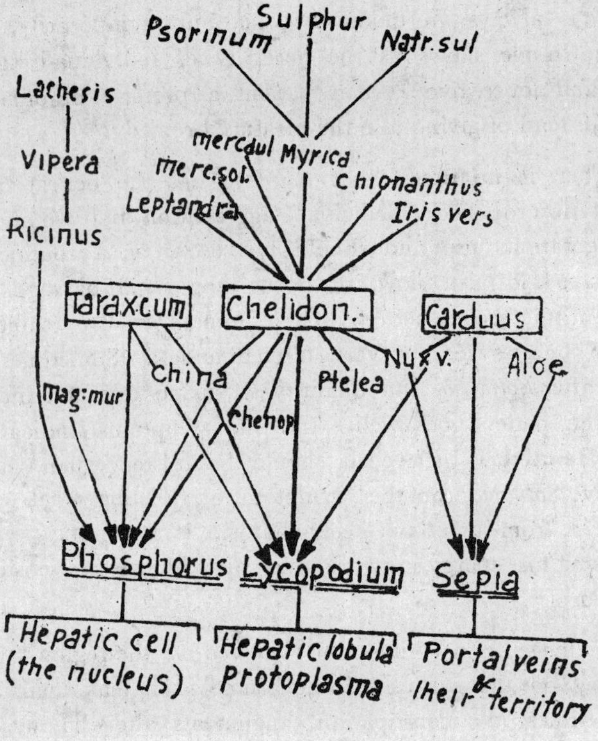

Relation of
TARAXACUM, CHELIDONIUM Lycopodium

F Bernoville

We must understand well the action of these medicines of drainage on the liver, because it is their action on the hepatic cells, on the liver itself allows a drainage either towards digestive apparatus, or to the urinary tract.

Imagine to yourself a hepatic lobula. The central veine of this lobula, the lobula itself with its hepatic cells, really called biliary ducts to the periphery. When you use some cholagogs, you act on the biliary ducts *i.e.* to say on the peripheric part of the lobula; *Phosphorus* in high dilutions given to a person suffering from insufficient liver, act on the liver, the blood and the kidneys. It is for this reason that *Phosphorus* is an important remedy of grave insufficient liver and of uremia. As regards the biliary ducts, *Lycopodium* and *Sulphur* will be more specially indicated. *Lycopodium* is a double edged arm; the more you give it in lower dilutions the more it will act on the periphery; the more you give it in high dilutions, the more it will come nearer to *Phosphorus*. This will help us to understand the chart. On this schema we have put *Chelidonium*, *Taraxacum* and *Carduus marianus* on the left lobe. Schematically, we may say that *Lycopodium*, *Phosphorus* and *Sepia* are the important ground remedies of these three remedies of drainage. *Solidago* being the drainage remedy of our whole chart.

Chelidonium. It is a remedy of drainage of the digestive apparatus although at first it creates constipation. But it has later on a very mild action on the liver and helps it to act slowly on the digestive apparatus. *Carduus marianus* constipates less than *Taraxacum* and helps us to get a rapid drainage acting on the constipation. For this reason, you may very well give to the same person to allay the constipation of *Chelidonium*, this remedy and *Taraxacum* alternately. But together they do not go very well.

The big *Chelidonium* grows in humid ditches, on old walls, in uncultivated places, ruins of rocks. It has alone, among the three remedies, the symptom : Aggravation by every change of weather. It may therefore be indicated in hydrogenoids and in some cases, *Chelidonium* may have for its ground remedies, *Natrum sulphuricum* or *Thuja.*

The big Chelidonium is used by the empirics for the treatment of epithelioma. What is interesting to recall here, is that it contains some alcaloids, chelidoni acid. These alcaloids and this acid have some narcotic properties analogous to those of papaverine. Both belong to the family of papavericae ; this fact explains that often a person, who will die of uremia, will pass through the stage of *Chelidonium,* before arriving to that of *Opium*. *Chelidonium* is a shaded off *Opium.*

Chelidonium has action on the skin ; it is used in the treatment of warts, because it is sufficiently caustic.

Elective Local Action. On an anatomical region. It is not only a remedy which acts on the right lobe but also on the lower part of the hemi-thorax (right) and on the right portion of the right hypochondria which includes the right lobe of the liver, the lower base of right lung, the right pleura in the same region and accessorily on the right thorax. It is for this reason *Chelidonium* is sometimes given in intercostal herpes.

You see here an example of a remedy which does not only act as tisane or on an organ but on a topographic region and according to metameric distribution. It acts on the right portion of the abdomen ; it is therefore a remedy of the right angle of the colon, of the right base of the right lung in some broncho-pneumonias and pneumonias of the right base.

You remember that it acts on the mucous membranes like *Hydrastis*, specially on those of the biliary apparatus, on the intestinal mucosa and finally it has a secondary action on the kidneys, the knees and on the occiput. A patient of *Chelidonium* may come to you for his headache on the occiput. You may, in that case think of a liver which is not working well and prescribe *Chelidonium* or *Juglans cineria.* In this case often the ground remedy is *Lachesis* : vertigo, pain of the occiput, gushes of heat, delayed menses or less abundant menses. *Lachnantes* may act electively if there is a rheumatism of the cervical vertebrae.

Action on the knees makes it related to *Cocculus*. Some patients of arthritis, whose liver works bad, have rheumatism specially of the knees : *Chelidonium*, *Cocculus*, *Bryonia and Symphytum*. The ground remedy will be *Natrum Muriaticum and Thuja* insufficient liver, arthritis, bad circulation. The toxins are not burnt, toxinic deposition on the articulations. If there is any intra-articular localisation : *Bryonia*. If there are extra-articular localisations : *Rhus tox*. With osteo-cartilagenous lesions : *Symphytum*. Cracklings in the knees, often with a liver that does not work well, with nausea in a coach or in a train *Cocculus*.

Do no forget that the vertigo of *Chelidonium* is related to the liver. The tongue is completely yellow, having imprint of the teeth (Mercurius and Hydrasis)

In *Chelidonium* : Aggr. by movement, change of climate by touch, cough, the north-east wind ; from 4 to 8 p.m. in the evening according to the elimination of urea in the urine.

Do not forget also its relation with *Arsenic Album* as both like heat, inverse of *Phosphorus*.

From practical point of view I like *Chelidonium* as a remedy of *Indigestion*. When a child or an adult has indigestion caused by fatty foods, it is a mervellous remedy like *Antimonium crudum* and *Nux vomica* with which you may give it alternately. The patient complains of his stomach while it is the liver which is affected.

Carduus Marianus. This plant grows in humid places, on the sides of the streets and on ruins. Men rerely eat it. However in some countries where there is famine, people eat this plant.

It is a very bitter plant and as such according to the doctrine of signatures it will act on the liver. This is possible because empirically it is said that the bitter plants act on the liver and on the bile. *Carduus* is used in precancer stage with high blood pressure. It acts on the liver specially on the left lobe, in jaundice, and empirically on leucorrhoea.

Local Elective Action. *Liver,* veins, specially portal veins (Sepia) while *Sulphur* acts on arterial and venous circulation of the abdomen. *Nux vomica* and *Aloe* act equally on portal veins ; *Carduus* has a general action on the venous system.

It acts secondarily on the mucous membranes, occiput, kidneys and on the knees but much less than *Chelidonium.*

The liver is big, often with vomitting of bile.

Amelioration by discharge of blood, agg. by lying on the left side and by beer like that of *Aloe.*

It seems to act not only on the liver but also on supra-renals specially the left one.

Pre-sternal pigmentation of the skin. This pigmentation in some subjects denotes a diminution of vital force, with supra-renal insufficiency and hepatic insufficiency premonitory symptom of cancer. It is often an important remedy of female genital cancer.

Taraxacum. This plant grows in the meadows, pasture grounds and on street sides. Cows, goats and sheeps feed on them and the bees like very much its flowers. We take it sometimes with salads. It grows on sandy grounds.

Empirically it is said that it is purifier and a tonic but Leclerc says that it is a double edged arm. It may excite or depress and it has been researched what was the number of blood globules before giving M.T. of *Taraxacum* in high doses ; it was seen that at the begining the number of hematies increases and that very soon, in the second stage the number diminishes. Therefore there is produced at first an excitation and then a depression.

Taraxacum with *Phosphorus* and *Kali Carbonicum* acts electively *on the supernumerary element of the blood. Kali carbonicum* is a remedy that we give in pre-hepatic dyspeptic troubles. This is an ordinary liver in sufficiency for which *Taraxacum* is an excellent drainage remedy.

Taraxacum contains Calcium, Sodium and Potassium (*Calcarea carbonica, Natrum muriaticum, Kali carbonicum*).

Among its characteristics let us insist on the *Mapped* tongue. It is the mirror of all the mucous membranes of the digestive apparatus. It is very difficult to explain it. As in *Natrum Muriaticm,* one may only say that there is bad elimination on the mucous membranes with often a tendency to blockage of the mucous membranes.

A remedy of pre-cancer or pre-uremic stage.

Local Elective Action. 1. On the *Liver*, medial lobe, billiary ducts. It is centrifugal because it acts on the central lobe of the liver.

2. On the tongue, blood, hematies.

3. Action on the sternocleidomastoids, that have contractions.

The ground remedies are *Lycopodium, Phosphorus, Thuja.*

Taraxacum is often a remedy of nuralgia. It acts on the knees but its action is not of any great importance as a local elective action.

Aggr. by rest, sitting or standing.

Amel. by walking and touch.

There may be an abdominal meteorism which makes it related to *China.* You may give to *Phosphorus* patient *China 30* and *Taraxacum 3x.*

Much night-sweats, a sign of cutaneous elimination.

Taraxacum seems to bring back a digestive elimination and stops vesical elimination.

An important remedy of indigestion with vomitting of hepato-biliary origin.

Dr. A. Nebel has taught me the application of *Peucedenum* when in the case of an aeorophagia with pyloro-duodenal syndrom, it is necessary to open the renal barrage, when the kidneys are blocked.

Hydrastis. It is really a type of medicine of universal drainage, like *Solidago* and *Berberis.* We think of it not only as a drainer of the digestive apparatus, but also of respiratory, genetary, and even urinary systems when it is the question of drainage through any mucous membranes and gland.

One of the most important characteristics is to produce a *Discharge of Mucous Extremely thick, Yellowish, Ropy, Tenacious and Adherent.*

Its another characteristic is *debility and weakness.* Hydrastis comes from Canada and we have only few ideas about its empiric use. It was first used by the homoeopaths. It is always the local elective action which makes it a remedy of drainage and canalisation. Action *Hydrastis* is as follows :

1. Action on the tissues which is very important. Surface action on mucous membranes. On tissues of which the value s schematised by two dimensions and not by three dimensions. Mucous of the stomach, biliary ducts, intestines. Secondarily on the uterine mucous membranes, then on the urethra; finally cavum and the *pharynx* more than on the bronchial mucous membranes.

2. The really elective action is produced on the *Stomach,* the *Biliary ducts, intestines, cavum* and the *pharynx.* The typical characteristic symptom is always, thick, yellow and thready discharge.

The discharge of *Hydrastis* is very similar to that of *Kali bichromicum* which is sometimes more corrosive than that of *Hydrastis*.

The discharge of any mucous membrane happens in this way :

1st Stage. Less abundant, fluid, less coloured and very corrosive of the type of *Arsenicum, Mercurius cor.* and *Nitric acid* (mixed with blood)

2nd Stage. Less abundant, thicker, becomes coloured, yellowish or greenish, adherent, ropy, thready.

3rd Stage. Abundant, thick, but non-corrosive (*Pulsatilla*)

It seems that in the first stage there is some toxic subsances because of the corrosiveness of the discharge. This gradually diminishes as the discharge continues and the mucous membrane is repaired.

Hydrastis can also be compared with an important remedy, *Kreosotum*, of which the flow is fluid, often mixed with blood like *Arsenic* or *Nitric acid*, excessively corrosive. The most important fact is that when you give one of these remedies, the corrosiveness of the discharge disappears very rapidly and you come to *Pulsatilla*. When there is no flow *Sulphur* is indicated or when the patient becomes a chronic one, *Silicea*, a remedy of fistula.

The action of *Hydrastis* is extremely variable according to the dilution used. We must know very well this medicine and we must have experience about its application, like *Kali bichromicum* and *Pulsatilla*, centrifugal in lower dilutions and centripetal in high and medium dilutions. It is rather from the 30th it stops the discharge. We must take care of this fact because when you give *Hydrastis* for a longtime in lower dilutions you may hasten the patient towards chronicity and towards fistula.

It may again be compared with *Kali sulphuricum*, the chronic of *Pulsatilla*, of which the discharge is the same, thick, mild, non-irritant.

On digestive apparatus, *Hydrastis* may act on two or three opposit poles. It is then a very interesting remedy of morbid metastasis, as for example.

—*Biliarg duct→cavum→pharynx.*

—*Biliary duct*→uterus

—*Uterus→cavum→pharynx.*

It is then a remedy of women who have white discharge, gonococcic or not, because of metritis. She goes to a specialist who cauterises her col uteri. Sometime after the operation she has rhino-pharingitis or an other affection of the *pharynx*; still it is a remedy of persons suffering from chronic hepatic troubles, who will gradually weaken his stomach and his intestine as a consequence of bile insufficiency and will latter on have rhino-pharyngitis with thick, yellow discharge from the *cavum* to the behind of the nose.

In the first stage it is preferable to give *Hydrastis* in low dilutions in order to favour the discharge and to cause a real drainage. One or two months after, when your patient is really well drained, when the discharge is no more irritating, you may give *Hydrastis* in high dilutions. One should never act in a centripetal sense on a corrosive discharge. On the contrary you are right to act in this way in cases of fistula or when the discharge is chronic and interminable which is the effect of the *Law of least effort.*

The action of *Hydrastis* on biliary ducts, as we have said, is externaly important. It gives good results, in lower dilutions in persons who had hepatic colic, not because they had an obstruction of the bile ducts by a stone, but because that obstruction was due to stopper in the choledoc (bile duct) which causes an icterus by retention and by spasm.

Really speaking it is a secondary remedy of hepatic colic. We have other more important remedies, first of all of the pain and then of deeper action on the hepatic cell : *China*, *Chionathus*, *Chelidonium*.

The works of Brule have shown that in icterus, even infectious and benign, there is always affection of the hepatic cell. In a word there always exists an acute stage. The retention is secondary, however, *Hydrastis* is to be considered in persons suffering from insufficient liver of ripe or of old age. It should be given after the age of fifty. It will also be prescribed in chronic dyspepsia, with diminution of gastric motility and of the secretion; persons who lose weight and who feels very much tired. They doubt the beginning of a cancer, or the cancer is already there. By treating them homoeopathically, it is seen that they put on weight, specially when Hydrastis is given. The patient seems to have arrived at cholecystitis and cancer of the stomach or of the intestines, with secondary metastasis towards the liver. Hydrastis acts specially at the time-limit.

Modalities. Aggr. by inspiration of cold air in dry weather, in open air and in a room with open windows, by slight discharge of blood.

It is a pre-cancer remedy and of suspected cancer, specially of the col uteri.

Hydrastis and *Sanicula* act well together in constipation.

Hydrastis acts specially on the cancer of mucosa with debility and secretion, that become very thick, or when the digestive function becomes very much defective. But it does not act so to say on the element tumour. It will act preferably at the moment of ulceration that preceeds tumour, callous ulcer which becomes cancer.

Condurango. It is used on the element tumour (stomach and pylora). It has a very important symptom : It defends by a contraction localised under the umbilical, right or left.

It is perhaps the most faithful of all the cancer remedies and it may be given in all possible dilutions. I prescribe it often in 200 followed by a 6 and by *Psorinum*. But for the latter one should not go beyond 30, to avoid any risk of aggravation.

In *Carbo animalis* the tumour is completely formed, and is very hard. There may be burning pain as if from a burning charcoal, which makes it related to *Arsenicum album*.

Conium is also indicated in tumours, cancers, specially glandular but it is much more inconstant than the two other.

If you give *Hydrastis* in very low dilutions in some cases, it may cause loss of weight while favouring the discharge. On the contrary very often you will get mervelous result by using it in M.T. or as local application.

Taraxacum, *Carduus marianus* and *Chelidonium* form the group of medicines of insufficient liver which may also act on pre-cancer stage or on persons who are in the process of developping cancer. It is for this reason they are related to *Hydrastis*. They are medicines of less grave stage than that of the last one.

Let us add that *Hydrastis*, wher one has well understood it, has a double action : Centrifugal in lower dilutions and centripetal in higher dilutions; it is a remedy which will help other inconstant remedies.

Chionanthus is a small remedy of drainage by the side of *Hydrastis*. If you search in the Materia medica for synthesising its action, you will see that it has local elective action only on two points : The *Liver* and the *Head*. I have discovered a third point, the *Pancreas* and I think that pancreatic insufficiency is a rule in *Chionanthus* and makes it related to *Iris versicolor*.

On the one hand it is the remedy of periodic bilious migraine, accompanied by vomitting, cold sweats (*Iris versicolor* and *Veratrum album*). The cold sweats are seen not specially on forehead like *Veratrum album* but also on the back of hands.

It has no doubt an action on the liver as it can produce jaundice. It is the remedy of all possible jaundices, of hepatic colics, of cholecystitis, of infections jaundice, or jaundice by retention of bile.

His diarrhoeic stools often contain undigested meat or small balls of fat, indicating not only hepatic insufficiency but also a pancreatic insufficiency.

Aggr. by movement and by cold.

Amel. while lying down on the belly (*Chelidonium* and *Sepia.*, *Kali carbonicum* is ameliorated by bending forward. *Bryonia* and *Colocynthis* are ameliorated by pressure and by bending double.

From the point of view of drainage, *Chionanthus* is a small remedy, however very constant of which the action may be schematised thus: very near to *Iris versicolor* as regards its periodic migraine, but it is a remedy of acute stage having important relation to the trio: *Mercurius* (solubilis or dulcis), *Chelidonium* and *China.*

In periodic migraines when *Iris versicolor* is indicated very often the ground remedies are *Natrum muriatium* or *Calcarea phos.*

You will then use *Cionanthus* in hepatic or bilious migraines, often with big, painful liver having tendency to jaundice with colourless stools, rather over coloured stools. It acts well in lower dilutions or in M.T. From the side of intestines it should not be used, to speak the truth as a drainer, but as a canaliser. It acts as a check when there is great hepatic insufficiency.

Myrica. It grows on marshy and uncultured lands of Western Europe and Cazin says that it is found in the suroudings of Versailles. It has a very strong smell, a bitter taste. The empirics say that it is a vermifuge, tonic, and excitant. It seems to contain a substance like hemp. It contains equally an oil which after decoration gives a product very near to wax, whence its name *Myrica serifera.*

Elective action on the heart and the *naso-pharynx.* It is really interesting to consider the number of remedies that act on the liver and at the sametime on *naso-pharynx.* It seems that the nasal discharge is a real supplementary outlet of drainage in subjects whose liver functions badly and whose digestive apparatus seems insufficint and this is seen more in men than in women. The intellectuals of the type of *Nux vomica,* specially the persons of sedentary habit who live in towns, who are aggr. by inhalation of dust, show the maximum frequency of rhino-pharingitis (chronic) which should always draw the attention on the genito-urinary system (Thuja type) or on the bad function of the liver.

In the **Materia Medica** we find in *Myrica* a discharge of thick and yellowish mucous which may cause nausea because of the effort to expectorate.

It is also sometimes, like *Chamomilla,* a remedy of jaundice. *Myrica* is very near to *Chionanthus* and *Chelidonium.* But there is a depressive action on the heart which is not found in *Chelidonium,* and very less in *Chamomilla.* It is for this reason related to *Digitalis.*

You know that in Jaundice, there may be slow pulse and a depressive action by the intermediary of the vagus on the cardiac muscles. This action is found in Myrica, but not so much as in Digitalis, palpitations and even cardiac weakness with hypotension. The liver is big and sometimes also the spleen.

Phosphorus, China and *Digitalis* form the trio of cardiac liver, of the accordeon liver; by asystole it becomes big by simple congestion, which may, later on, cause cardiac cirrhosis, with secondary degeneration of the *parenchyma* of the type of *Phosphorus*. In such cases one should not give only *Digitalis* in ponderable doses, because of its mechanical action on the myocardia but one should know how to use Digitalis in homoeopathic dilutions. Even in 30 and 200 it may give wonderful results. When the symptoms of *Digitalis* are found on the heart alone, use *Digitalis* in gross doses or even use maceration of its leaves, but when the heart symptoms are related to liver in an asystolic patient whose balance is more or less unstable with a big liver one should raise the dilution of *Digitalis*.

You may often have to prescribe as for example *Phosporus* 200, followed by *China* 30, *Digitalis* 30 and *Digitalis* Ix. In such a case *Myrica* becomes a small supporting remedy. I do not know whether it has an action on the respiratory system, because I never use it alone. But it seems that it re-enforces the action of other remedies.

Berberis. A hepatic drainer, may also be considered with other drainers of the urinary system.

It is a plant of our country, that is found in hedges and forests, near farms. It is a thorny plant of which the fruits are red. The sheeps and lambs breed on it.

The empirics recommend it in the liver diseases, in hydropsy and in dysenteries.

Leclerc, in his "Treaties on phytotherapy", makes of it a bitter tonic, and it seems that its action on the urinary system is not well known. With the berries of Berberis, in some honey, they prepare a special hydromel, somewhat tasteful to drink which has an acidulated flavour and which acts strongly on the urinary apparatus.

We have said that Hydrastis is for us a drainage type of mucous membranes; that *Solidago* is a typical drainage remedy of the liver towards digestive and urinary apparatus; Berberis is for homoeopaths, the typical remedy for fighting against metastasis and it is necessary to use it in relation to ground remedies, to check the transfer of the disease.

By making some analysis it is found, in Berberis, there are two cristalisable substances: The Berberine, and Maril or hydric acid.

Homoeopathic action of Berberis. Very great pains,very acute, in the abdomen or in the lumber region, liver and kidney. They have always clear-cut character of *Irradiating* along the urethra.

Modalities: Aggr. by movements, jerkings, standing, walking, specially while walking rapidly and with jerking steps. (One should think of this remedy when a patient says that he feels bad in a bus). He is aggravated after fatigue and after micturition.

Elective Local Action. On the *Kidney*, on the *Bladder*, on the *Digestive tract*. While the empirics know its action on the liver, they do not know its action on the kidney and we know that its primary action is on the urinary apparatus. It has besides an action on the lumber region, on the whole perineal region so as to become not only a remedy of nephritic colics but even a remedy of lumbago. Its action extends even to hips. Here we find, like *Chelidonium* that topographic action of homoeopathic remedies goes beyond the organ itself.

I may add that Berberis has undeniable action on the skin. When it is the question about this remedy we must think of the three important ways of elimination: liver, kidney and skin. Berberis is a remedy of which the intoxication produces very rapidly some pains while irritating with a hepatic congestion and almost always uricemia or azotemia. The blood undergoes some changes and this is why Berberis is, to be sure, a remedy of urticaria, a prelude to azotemia under the influence of an insufficient liver.

In this case the person who should normally eliminate by the liver and kidneys is obliged to find out a third way of elimination. *Berberis* aggr. the itching and sometimes causes the reappearence of an eruption like *Sulphur*, *Arsenicum*, *Lycopodium*. The important ground remedies of which *Berberis* is the complementry: Thuja and *Lycopodium*. And these two remedies are precisely the remedies of pre-uremic stage and of uremia. *Lycopodium*, has primordial action on the liver, and on the kidney. With *Thuja*, you act on the kidneys without aggravating the cutaneous symptoms, while *Berberis* seems to be related in this case to *Lycopodium*. When you give it one would say that the kidney is relatively relieved by causing eruption on the skin. This causes a good effect on condition that it is not exaggeraged. On my part, I have often seen that in insufficient liver it seems to drain much better *Phosphorus*, than *Lycopodium*, because, *Lycopodium* has already the tendency to drain through the skin. *Berberes* is the link from the point of view of polarity, the liver and the kidney and accessorily the skin It is the remedy-type when it is necessary to eliminate by the classic remedy that homoeopaths use and which is very difficult to prescribe. I think that it is not so faithful, though sometimes it gives marvelous results. Sometimes on the contrary it has some after effects. It acts remarkably well when used externally in M. T. as compresses.

We have therefore the interest to use *Berberis* to persons who are capable of urinary discharges, and in this regard one may compare it with *Magnesia borocitrica* and *Pardera brava*, specially in nephritic colic. *Fragaria* in urtericaria, *Urtica urens* is quite near to *Berberis* by its action on urticaria and by the drainage of urates through urines.

From the hepatic point of view, it has some relation to *Magnesia muriatica* and sometimes to *Hydrastis*. From urinary point of view with : *Coccus cacti*, *Terebinthina*, when the urines are red, rare and there is dysuria.

To check the aggr. of ***Berberis*** on the skin you may give the drainage remedy of A. Neble : ***Fumaria*** and ***Saponaria***, 10 gtts of lx which act remarkably canalising ***Berberis*** avoiding eczema and the itchings.

China naturally is an important medicine of hepatic insufficiency which I cannot describe in detail for want of space. You will find all its indications in the Materia Medica. You know that this is the first remedy experimented by Hahnemann. Really speaking it is not a ground remedy because it does not act very well in very high dilutions and as a remdy of temperaments, but it is indicated in all sorts of troubles and it acts electively on the liver and the blood, on all losses of organic fluids and haemorrhages. ***It is an importaut remedy of Centripetal Action and in this it opposes our important Centrifugal Sulphur.*** It is for this reason it should be given with great precaution because it may aggravate by blockage. However, as we have said, it plays an important part in the drainage or to be exact it helps us to make derivations.

China is very often, hypercholesterinemic and hydrogenoid. I have already spoken of these ***China*** types of cholesterinemics who are swollen with water and who really are dehydrated because the water that they have in their tissues cannot be used by them. They are used by the cholesterin which is very avid of water. The water behaves in human organism like a foreign body which does not serve to the exchanges and rather does not have any service in the intracellular life. What is characteristic of life and which shows well the action of the important homoeopathic remedies, such as ***Natrum Muriaticum*** and ***China***, is this balancing, of these exchanges that are done between the intracellular spaces and intercellular spaces. The young subject, full of life, has some hydrophile cells; the subject who advances in age, gradually as he is more and more used up has more and more hydrophobic cells and the retention of water; in persons of advanced age who become hydrogenoid or carbo-nitrogenoid in the intercellular space; the dehydration, the demineralisation and the loss of life are caused in the cells themselves. Whereas in subjects who are still young and who have a powerful life, the cells are hydrophobic, swollen with water; it is for this reason, the children have thirst very often because they have the need to ingest water necessary for their intracellular exchanges.

China is an important regulator of intercellular spaces with *Natrum sulphuricum*, while *Natrum muriaticum* in high dilutions is a regulator of intracellular spaces. *Natrum Muriaticum* acts on the intercellular spaces when it is given in lower dilutions in triturationts

COLOCYNTHIS, DIOSCOREA VILLOSA, BRYONIA BELLADONNA, CHAMOMILLA.

These are the five remedies of painful spasms of the biliary ducts. They act also electively on the *cross road* (right) of the colon (spasms, adherences, pericholecystitis, pericolitis) .

All the five are important remedies of hepatic colic.

In order to act soon these remedies should not be used internally alone (6 preferably) but also externally, local use of a compress of hot humid flannel on which should be sprinkled 5 to 10 drops of one or many of these drugs in alcoholatures (M. T.)

Dioscorea villosa and *Colocynthis*, both are important remedies, oppose one another.

Dioscorea villosa. The pain obliges the patient to stretch and even to bend backwards. Irradiation of the pain from the gall bladder to the back, to arms, to heart and specially to the *right breast.*

The pain appears suddenly. It is localised, *on some very definite points* and which may be covered by the finger tip.

Rumblings. Emission of gas. Flatulence (specially in tea drinkers). Better by walking. Heart beat is weak. Protruding hemorrhoids.

General aggravation in the evening, at night, while lying down, by bending forward. Amel. by stretching, and by pressure.

It is indicated in hepatic colic more than *Colocynthis.*

Colocynthis. *Pain better by bending double* and *Hepaiic* pressing strongly the belly. *Colic after anger*. Pain often localised in the umbilical region.

Colocynthis acts more on calculus lying more below than *Dioscoria*. Cramping pain, cramps are more marked in *Colocynthis*, *Amel*. by heat.

Bryonia. It is hardly indicated in the books. It has never given me good results. It suits to hepatic colic, which makes the patient immobile while nephritis requires movement.

Bryonia is complementary to *Diosboreia*, is amel. by pressure, having a very localised pain. But that pain is pricking and amel/by rest, whereas *Dioscorea* may often aggr. by rest and by lying down. These two remedies may be alternated. They help each other and do not antidote. In *Bryonia* : thirst for cold water. Liver is often big and congested ; *Amelioration of pain by Lying down on the painful side* Nausea and vomiting. Aggr. by movement, while sitting up or by standing up on the bed. The stomach is sensitive to touch. Pressure in the stomach as if by a stone. Frequent fever.

Belladonna, is related to *Colocynth*. It is very spaomodic , aggr. of pain by the least jerk, by the least touch. Extreme sensitiveness to touch. Face red, dilated pupils. Frequent fever. Sweats.

Chamomilla. Hepatic pain after anger with great irritability, capriciousness, never satisfied. Aggr. at night, and by the heat. Flatulence, distension of the abdomen. Fever with one cheek red the other pale and cold.

Podophyllum, Aloe, Aescuslus hippocastum and Collinsonia.

These are the four remedies of portal hypertension and of hemorrhoids or rectal troubles having relation to hepatic manifestations.

Podophyllum. It enters into all possible laxatives of the official medicine. It is considered to have an important action on the intestines.

Here is as we understand its effects in homoeopathy. Before all *it has a local elective action on the rectum* and secondarily *action on the duodenum* and thirdly a less important action on *the small intestines.*

Podophyllum therefore acts as you see on the two extremities of the intestines ; duodenum and rectum and its action on the duodenum is divided into two by an action on the biliary duct and the liver. It creates a motion for stools because it forces the gall bladder to empty itself. When the bile enters into the intestines it accelerates the intestinal transit. The reflex action of the bile causes strong contractions of the intestines. One is tempted to believe that it has no action on the stomach and consequently it cannot acts on the first portion of the duodenum. But podophyllum acts well on the duodenum, more particularly on the second and third portion of the duodenum, specially on the second and the third portion of Vater's ampula to the anastomosis of the *Choledochous* canal.

We have said that the action on the rectum is the most important. But *Podophyllum* may have a secondary action on the right ovary, on the right scapula and on the right side of the pharynx. You see then it has a rightsidedness. All the regions of its action are on the right of the axis of the human body.

Modalities. Aggravation in the morning towards 5 a.m. (diarrhoea forcing the individual out of the bed) ; while eating, during dentition, by drinking, by movement and by mercurial treatment.

Amelioration : Lying on the belly.

The diarrhoea of *Podophyllum* is accompanied by gurglings, profuse stools, putrid, without pain, very abundant, noisy and of clear yellow colour.

The colour of the stools should be kept in mind. Really the stools are colourless because of the absence of bile. Acholia. They are noisy because of gas, putrid and very foetid because of the want of bile to disinfect the fecal matter. Finally the stools are painless (*Phosphoric a.c. Kali bich.*). You know that it suits to infantile cholera. The prolapsus of the rectum, during dentition and in summer. Kent insists much on Podophyllum in his Materia Medica because it is the remedy that converted him to homoeopathy ; he had a patient whose diarrhoea was extremely foetid, putrid, and have obnoxious smell and he obtained a very good result by *Podophyllum.*

The diarrhoea of *Arsenic* is also very foetid but blackish. *Arsenicum* is a good remedy of food poisoning, ptomain poisoning and poisoning by all other foods which are not fresh; the putridity is even cadaveric.

Relation of Podophyllum. A group of medicines of drainage of the digestive apparatus are complementaries and are of the first importance with a ground remedy *Sulphur.* The group is : *Nux vomica, Argentum nitricum, Anacardium. Aloe, Aesculus hippocastum, Podophyllum, Magnesia sulphurica* and all the Mercuries are related to *Sulphur.*

Mercurius dulcis, Mercurius solubilis and Mercurius corrosivus act on the whole digestive system, specially on the mouth, on the duodenum, liver, pancreas, intestines and *Mercurius corrosivus* on the rectum.

Argentum nitricum acts electively on the stomach and duodenum and secondarily on the small intestines. In mucomembranous enteritis it is related to two other remedies : *Cupressus* and *Cantharis,* All the three act on the bladder.

Anacardium acts on the stomach and duodenum, secondarily on the intestines. It has also an action on the skin ; the liver and on the mind.

Nux vomica. It is an important polychrest which is however, a drainer and complementary of *Sulphur.* It is, says

Dr. Nebel, the canaliser of *Sulphur* on the small intestines in acute conditions. When you have indigestion with diarrhoea then constipation, then again diarrhoea, it is indicated. It regulates the peristaltism of the small intestines and *Nux Vomica*, says Huge-Saxons, is the remedy of debauchery.

Aloe is the canaliser of *Sulphur* on the rectum.

Aesculus hippocastum has a special action on portal hypertension and on the veins of the rectum (Sepia)

Magnesia sulphuricum is the most active remedy to empty the gall bladder. It is a cholagog type.

Podophyllum is equally near to *China* as regards diarrhoea, at first bilious, then devoid of bile. Through *China* it is related to *Phosphorus* with its great hepatic insufficiency.

It has equally relation, either direct or through *Bryonia*, with *Natrum muriaticum*, a remedy of chronic stage which in an acute stage yields its place to *Podophyllum*.

From the point of view of drainage, the application of *Podophyllum* is interesting, but it should not be used in very high dilutions because it blocks very soon. Better use it in the 6th. It is a complementing remedy of functional nature because of its centripetal tendency, rather than a drainage remedy properly called. It is also a canaliser because of its action on the two poles : *Duodenum* and *rectum*.

Aloe. A very interesting remedy. At first it acts electively on the rectum, less on the liver, colons and on the whole large intestine.

From the anatomical point of view it acts on the lumber region, on the pelvis, and on the female genitals.

On veins from the point of view of tissues.

Its action on the liver should not be neglected. The action is sufficiently strong. Hepatic insufficiency with portal hypertension very marked. Generalised venous congestion, localised specially on the abdomen and on the portal system.

You know the important symptoms of *Aloe*. Weakness of the sphinister which causes incontineunce when passing air. Tendency to prolapsus of the anus like *Podophyllum*.

Aloe then should be used in the diarrhoea according to the law of homoeopathy. It is to be given in 30. It is a very important remedy because of its local elective action on the rectum, and it is a drainage remedy. While *Podophyllum* is almost always centripetal in homoeophathic doses, *Aloe* may be centrifugal in medium dilutions.

When the symptoms of *Aloe* is very marked, while the diarrhoea is only transitory or even non-existent *Aloe* may be an excellent remedy of constipation due to the rectal atony having portal congestion. Dr. William Bas gives it daily with *Taraxacum* in old chronic constipated persons. The allopaths who give *Aloe* and *Podophyllum* in massive doses soon fatigues the liver causing colourless stools with acholia and overwork of the liver which can no more secrete the bile.

We must also know that *Aloe* is a remedy to be given to old beer drinkers having aggr. by beer like *Kali bichromicum*. Dr. A. Nebel who has well studied *Aloe*, says that it acts on oxalemic persons specially more than on uratics, but no experimental researches have yet been done on this point.

Aggravation by Beer. *Kali bichromicum* is very important. *Aloe* is often the remedy of old persons. Note here that persons who have atony of the rectum are either old or child. An old man who has great atony of the rectum with constipation, may have complete atony of the anal sphinister with constipation, like that of the type of *Causticum*.

Aggravation by Wine. *Nux Vomica* is an important remedy. But you may have other remedies : *Zincum metallicum* and *Antimonium crudum*. The last one is very much aggravated by sour wine. As regards *Zincum* wine makes it terribly restless. Tremblings, spasms, restlessness of the legs.

Sulphur is the ground remedy of all these persons when they drink too much wine, beer or coffee. They have high blood pressure with congestive symptoms.

Aggravation by Coffee or Tea. *Ignatia.* Less important are *Chamomilla* and *Gelsemium*. *Aconite* is very much indicated in persons who cannot tolerate Cafeine. In these cases *Adrenalin* in the 30th and 200th will also act. Coffee decafeined, may be tolerated by these subjects.

In aggravation by tea one may use *Selenium* which is also used in sexual excesses and for the throat, the liver. Another important remedy is *Thuja.*

Already towards 1848, Hering had shown that the people generally, drink beer, drink also tea, and that those who consume a large quantity of coffee drinks too much wine because coffee antidotes the action of wine to some extent and the tea antidotes the effects of beer. Coffee has a good reaction after meals when the wine has caused some troubles. On the other hand one should note that in persons who cannot tolerate tea, there is extreme dilatation of the stomach. Give them *Thuja.*

When the subject is intoxicated by cocaine give him *Gelsemium* and a cup of coffee if it is necessary.

Aggravation by Tobacco. *Gelsemium*, *Ignatia*, *Nux vomico*, *Daphne indica*, *Caladium*, *Plantago.*

Aesculus Hippocastum. Action on the *rectum*, the right side of the abdomen and secondarily on the liver and the pharynx. It may also acts on mucous membranes, occiput and on the lumber region. The same action on the occiput like that of *Juglans cineria.*

Modalities. Aggr. in the morning after waking up, walking, after stools and micturition.

Amelioration. In open air, by cold bath, by the discharge of blood from haemorrhoids, continued exercise.

Aesculus is an important complementary of *Sulphur*. But when you have a patient of *Sulphur* having portal congestion, when haemorrhages from the haemorrhoids are not painful, it is the history of the subject who maintains a good health because he has periodic haemorrhages from the haemorrhoids; the bleeding is natural and it is good for health. Sometimes this haemorrhage may stop; he becomes aggravated, has the sensation of a plug with pins in the rectum or a bit higher in. Very often when you examine a patient you may find that he has the symptoms of *Sulphur* and of *Aesculus* as well. He is in a period of transition. He will have his prescription in the following manner ***Sulphur 200***, ground remedy, ***Nux vomica** 30*, functional remedy, to act on the constipation and on genaral congestion; *Aesculus* 3, 6, or 30 the drainer and at the same time the derivator which will diminish the portal congestion, stop the haemorrhoidery derivation. The patient will drain himself either through the skin or by urine. Thus you will help the digestive system.

Relation. *Podophyllum*, *Aloe*, *Nux vomica*, *Chamomilla* (intolerence to pain), *Belladonna*. The last two make it related to *Calcarea carbonica* and thus brings it nearer to *Sulphur*. *Aesculus* is also related to *Coffee*. From the point view of the throat, it has other important relations than in the affection of *Pharynx*. It is often complementary to *Phytolacca*, *Hamamelis*, *Kali muriaticum* and *Arsenic*.

Collinsonia. Less important than the preceding three. A remedy of drainage acting electively on the rectum but specially on the entire pelvis, uterus, intestines and on the colons. Secondarily on the liver and on the pharynx.

Haemorrhoids specially in time of pregnancy. Pelvic congestion with varicocele. Burnning pain of the rectum. Cardiac pains, constipation. Bleeding piles alternating with cardiac troubles and rheumatism.

Often a *Pulsatilla* woman becomes a patient of *Collinsonia*. *Collinsonia* has also relation with *Lycopodium*, *Nux vomica*, and *Sulphur*, distantly related to *Sepia*.

Modalities. Aggravation : at night specially, by sudden suppression of the haemorrhoids. It is a good remedy of derivation but when you use *Collinsonia*, on haemorrhoids be careful of the consequences. If you open the intestine, you naturally favour elimination through this organ but that will not be enough. You should very often give *Lycopodium* or *Thuja* as a ground remedy, *Nux vomica* as a functional remedy and *Solidago*, *Berberis* to open more the anal passage.

Always try to drain, to derivate through the kidney as much as possible for avoiding metastasis. And be careful, by suppressing the haemorrhoids, not to cause in the patient a liver headache.

On this subject we make a rapid comparison of the remedies of haemorrhoids.

I am not speaking again about *Sulphur*, which is well studied in the **Materia Medica** and about *Hamamelis* and *Nux vomica*, *Aloe* and *Aesculus*.

Very Painful Haemorrhoids : think of *Muriatic acid*, *Nitric acid*, *Poeonia*, *Ratanhia* (fissures)

Aesculus has the sensation of a plug with needles in the rectum and its haemorrhoids bleed little.

Muriatic acid has the sensation of excoriation. The haemorrhoids are very red, very much excoriated, so painful that when the patient goes to stool he is obliged to wipe with a damped cotton. It is also related to *Lachesis* which has also sensitiveness to touch. The whole mucous membrane is excoriated and infected.

Nitric Acid. It has the sensation that he is pricked by many needles. It has anal fissures.

There is pressure in *Poeonia* and *Ratanhia*.

There are two other remedies of painful haemorrhoids, often related to *Aesculus* : *Kali carbonicum* and *Ignatia.*

Kali carbonicum has "stitches", pricking by needles from below upwards. Amel. by pressure.

Ignatia has paradoxal symptoms.

The cases of the type of *Aloe* and of *Hamamelis* bleed much, have no great pains and for them you are forced to use *Arnica* and *China* for the bleeding. They have almost the necessity of bleeding from the piles. When their haemorrhoids are treated locally or suppressed by surgery, they may suffer from grave troubles, as for example cancer of the abdomen because their haemorrhoids are the outlet of drainage. *Sulphur* is the ground remedy of these patients who will later on suffer from cancer of the digestive apparatus. The patient, at the same time suffers from arterial and venous hypertention specially of the abdomen. He has gradually come down by the stages of *Lycopodium* and *Graphitis.* He arrived at a given time in the stage of *Sepia,* then of *Thuja.* From *Thuja* he passes to *Carbo animalis,* more than to *Carbo vegetabilis.* When the cancer is formed one should think of *Condurango, Hydrastis, Carbo animalis* but the condition has become already grave. If the patient was treated preventively, one could, by causing the hypertension, abdominal and portal, check the formation of cancer.

PTELIA LEPTANDRA JUGULANS CINEREA YUCCA FILAMENTOSA.

Four necessory remedies of hepato-biliary troubles.

Leptandra : Jaundice with painful liver and, *Abundant Stools, Hyperbilious, Black, like Foetid Coal Tar.*

Pain in the umbilical region extending from the liver to the vertebral column. Yellow tongue.

Better by lying down on the belly. Aggr. by drinking cold drinks, by movement and periodically. It may have like *Phosphorus*, haemorrhoids originating from the liver and protruding haemorrhoids bleeding very much.

The ground remedies to which *Leptendru* is related are *Phosphorus* and *Lachesis*. It also has some relations to *Baptisia, Arsenicum* and *Chionanthus*. *Leptandra* is one of the rare remedies of the Materia medica which has clear bilious stools, black and deep green, overcharged with bile. It suits to persons having insufficient liver whose gall-bladder and even the hepatic cells are blocked for a time, and who, at a given time, secrets a great quantity of bile in the intestines (*Mercurius*) may also have hyperbilious greenish stools.

Hyperbilious *Leptandra* opposes to *Chlidonium, Myrica, Chionanthus, China* and to other remedies having rather acholia, and hypocholia. Very few remedies have this particular symptom of *Leptandra.*

Jugulans Cineria is used in persons suffering from insufficient liver who have headache near the neck and occiput accompanied by liver troubles and sometimes pain in the right shoulder, like that of *Chelidonium* and also biliary lithiasis.

It is related to *Chelidonium,, Bryonia* and *Iris versicolor.*

Ptelia. It is a small remedy of liver, complementary to *Sepia.* It suits to insufficient liver *Aggravated by Lying on the right side.*

Gastric atony is seen. There is a frontal headache. Has relation with *Sepia, Magnesia muriatica. Nux vomica.* It is interesting to use it in portal hypertension with troubles due to *Sepia.*

It is a good complementary of *Sepia.*

(The author has not studied the remaining groups most possibly because they are already studied in the first part of the book.)

RECAPITULATIVE TABLE OF THE THERAPEUTICS OF LIVER.

GROUND REMEDIES.

Lycopodium. Remedy of bile; proteolysis, atrophy.

Phosphorus. Glycogenic function; hypertrophic "processus", degeneration (fatty).

Sulphur. Proteolysis; general excretion; hereditary tuberculinism.

Natrum sulphuricum. Big torpid liver; hepato-renal insufficiency, oedemas.

Lachesis. Alcoholic cirrhosis; asystole; infections, circulatory troubles.

Arsenicum album. Infectious hepatitis; grave cases.

Sepia. Circulatory troubles (portal); proteolytic function.

Nux vomica. Spasmodic troubles.

INSUFFICIENT LIVER.

(*a*) *BILIARY FUNCTION.*

1. Hypercholia. Mercurius solubilis and dulcis, Leptandra.

2. Hypocholia. China, Chelidonium, Podophyllum, Chionanthus ; Myrica (jaundice), Magnesia sulphuricum (in ponderable dose), Digitalis (heart).

3. Pains. Arnica, Carduus, Chamomilla (irritable), Colocynthis (amel. by bending double); Dioscoria (amel. by stretching); Magnesia phosphorica (cramp), Bryonia (aggr. by movement), Chelidonium,

(*b*) *GLYCOGENIC FUNCTION.*

Uranium nitricum, Syzizium, Cephalandra indica M.T. Eucailptus (infusion); Morus nigra (infusion), Sulphur.

C. PROTEOLYTIC FUNCTION.

Ammon carb (uremia), Urea, Berberis (boiling sensation in the renal region (Baryta muriatica (white stools, hypertension) Solidago (excess of uric acid) (uremia), Urtica (dissolves uric acid); Thlaspi bursa pastoris.

D. PROTEOLYTIC FUNCTION WITH ACETONEMIA.

Senna, Belladonna (alternate with Senna); Cuprum arsenicosum (ureic convulsions); Calcarea muriatica (acetonuria, vomiting).

E. ANTITOXIC FUNCTION

Arsenicum album (food poisoning, ptomain); Phosphorus (effects of anesthetics), China, Nux vomica (purgatives, medicine, coffee, alcohol); Antimonium crudum (indigestion); Zanziber (bread, melons); Colocynthis and Alumina (starch food, potato); Veratrum album (choleriform diarrhoea).

F. PROTEOPEXIC FUNCTION (anaphylaxis). Apis (oedema, bee stings); Ledum (melons); Diluted horse serum (30), Urtica M.T., Fragaria (urticaria).

G. BLOOD FUNCTION. Phosphorus (delayed coagulation); Lachesis (purpura) China.

CIRRHOSIS.

a. Sclerosis. Aurum muriaticum, Aurum metallicum, Plumbum, Silicea, Iodium, Arsenicum iodatum, Kali iod.

b. Syphilis. Mercurius with Aurum and Plumbum.

c. Induration. Graphitis, Taraxacum, Fluoric acid, Conium.

d. Fatty degeneration. Phosphorus, Kali bichromicum, Phlorizin, Vanadium, Picric acid.

e. Pigmentary. Argentum nitricum.

f. Cancer. Carduus, Taraxacum, Conium, Hydrastis. Cholesterinum.

g. Ascitis. Carduus, China, Seneceo, Apocynum. Digitalis, Acetic ac. Prunus.

CONGESTION.

a. Passive. Sulphur, Natrum sulphuricum, Phosphorus (cardiac liver), Digitalis, China, Podophyllum, Apocynum, Kali carbonicum.

b. Active (Paludism). China, Natrum muriaticum.

HEPATITIS

a. Beginning. Aconite, Bryonia, Chamomilla.

b. Developed. Mercurius, Chelidonium, Podophylum, Chionanthus, China, Nux vomica. Iris versicolor.

c. Chronic. The above mentioned remedies and Ammon muriaticum, Cholesterinum, Kali iodatum, Kali muriaticum, Kali bichromicum, Iodium, Hydrastis.

d. Grave cases. Vipera, Arsenicum album, Lachesis, Phosphorus.

e. Alcoholic. Nux vomica, Sulphuric acid. Ammonium muriaticum, Arsenicum, Absinthium, Fluoric acid.

f. Portal Hypertension. Aloe. Aesculus. Leptandra, Collinsonia, Sepia, Pulsatilla.

g. Splenomegalia. Ceanothus.

h. Some particular modalities.

Pain aggr. lying on the left : Ptelea, Bryonia, Natrum sulph.

Pain aggr. lying on the right side. Magnesia muriaticum, Mercurius, Chelidonium, Dioscoria, Kali carbonicum.

Aggr. by friction. Podophyllum.

Feeling of on-coming diarrhoea, mapped tongue, vesicular eruption. Rananculus, Sceleratus.

Gall Bladder. *Elective action. Phosphorus (M), with Lutein (200, M) Bryonia, Ricinus, Arsenicum album, Lachesis, Dioscorea, Chelidonium, Juglans, Natrum sulphuricum.*

Bile Ducts. *Hydrastis, Colocynthis, Chelidonium, Nux vomica, Magnesia muriatica.*

Right Lobe. *Chelidonium.*

Left lobe. Carduus.

Pancreas. *Phosphorus, Iris versicolor.*

Vater's ampouls. Mercurius dulsis, Lycopodium.

SMALL INTESTINES.

Pylora. Ornothagallum.

Duodenum. Kali bichromicum, Anacardium, Argentum nitricum

Intestines. Nux vomica, Graphitis, Sulphur, Ipecac, Cina, China, Croton, Veratrum album, Arsenicum album, Plumbum, Stannum, Opium.

COLON, Caecum. *Thuya, Ignatia, Bryonia.*

Ascending. Bryonia, Rhux tox.

Sigmoid. Kali bichromicum, Ipecac.

RECTUM AND ANUS. *Mercurius solubilis, Mercurius corrosivus, Aloe, Sepia, Podophyllum, Aesclus, Collinsonia, Silicea, Nitric ac, Fluoric acid, Sulphur.*

It need not be said that the above table should not be used mechanically. By doing so the doctors will face grave failures. It should be used as a "*mnemonics*" after a clinical examination and only when the diagnosis is done. With this reserve we may say that the above table will be useful.

GENERAL TABLE OF THE TREATMENT OF JAUNDICE

(Except hemolytic Jaundice)

Infectious and habitual icterus and retention of bile	*Other remedies of Jaundice*		*Grave forms*
Outset Aconite Bryonia Chamomilla *Established* Chelidonium Myrica Chionanthus China *Minerals.* Merc. cor, sol, dulcis *Urinary drainage* Berberis	*Infectious. Secondary remedies* Nux vomica Aloe Kali carb Kali bichr. Natrum phos. Nitric ac. Iodum Juglans cin *Pleochromatic jaundice* Leptandra Yuces *Infantile* Lupulus	*Jaundice with cirrhosis or precancer stage* Aurum mur. natr. Aurum metal. Plumbum Carduus marianus Taraxacum Hydrastis Conium Vipera Cholesterinum *Malarial janndice* China Ceanothus *Jaundice with pruritis plus* olichos pr.	*Serpents* *Crotalus* Lachesis Naja *Minerals* Phospherus Ars. alb Merc cor *Vegetables* *Typhoid type of fever* Gels., Baptisia Arnica; Rhus t. *Influenza type of fever.* Eupat perf Gelsemium Rhus t. Verat alb. *Action on gall bladder* Podo, Digitalis, China. *Other remedies* Hydrastis, Ceanothus.
Ground remedies	*Ground remedies.*		*Ground remedies*
Lycopodium Sulphur, Natrum sulph	Lpcopodium and Phosphorus Sulphur, Natrum sulph. Lachesis Natrum muriaticum, Sepia		Phosphorus Lachesis

JAUNDICE, BENIGNANT AND INFECTIOUS

Benignant infectious jaundice is caused by the penetration of microbes in the biliary ducts.

The infection may be of ascending origin (*Colibacilli, Eberth's bacillus*), or of sanguin origin and may be very frequent. It often happens that the hepatic infection is primary manifestation of infectious state and jaundice then seems to be primitive.

According to the seriousness of infection, we may have three varieties of benignant infectious jaundice.

1. Very benign infectious icterus, manifests itself by some digestive troubles, anorexia, thirst, nauseous condition, general weakness and uneasiness. Objectively a very slight icterus may be noted, which may be very clearly seen on the conjunctivas, temperature may remain normal.

2. Catarrhal Icterus. After prodromic phase of very benignant icterus, gradually clear symptoms of jaundice are seen. The tongue is white, bitter taste in the mouth, more or less discoloured stools, the urines are foamy, of mahogny colour and contains some salts and traces of albumin, the temperature rises from 38°C to 38.5°C for a few days. In spite of the temperature the pulse is slow. The liver and the spleen are slightly enlarged in volume. The skin may be the seat of intense pruritis.

3. If the condition aggravates still more, the temperature may rise from 30°C to 40°C there is chill, restlessness, head-ache, epistaxis. The liver as well as the spleen are voluminous. The urine is rare and abundant ; there is at the sametime azotemia. This conditions may remain from two to three weeks and the convalescence may begin with a change in the urine. This form always follows with a long convalescence with great emaciation. Infectious icterus with not a high temperature, at the beginning, is very difficult to differentiate

from grave icterus, having such a symptomatic picture. One must be very careful in his diagnosis.

In the presence of such and such clinical picture what remedies the homoeopath may think of ? We are going to pass them in review without being able to give a list for each of the varieties mentioned above, because the same remedy may be used in any one of the different cases. The remedies will be used according to the symptoms present.

Aconitum. Jaundice consecutive to a cold, fright, intestinal catarrh. Constant pain in the epigastric region irradiating to the naval region, or alternating from liver to stomach. Tongue coated thick and yellowish, constipation or diarrhoea. Fever with chill ; hard pulse, full, strong. Anxiety.

Berberis. Dry scaly tongue ; lancinating or pressive pain in the hepatic region, aggr. by pressure. Morbid appetite alternating with anorexia to food or great thirst alternating with dislike for any kind of drink. Constant uneasyness in the stomach which is full of wind, and from time to time emission of noisy gas. Pale stools, ashy grey, or profuse watery diarrhoea, irritant. Deep coloured urine, turbid with thick deposit.

Bryonia. Thick white coating of the tongue. Nausea, regurgitations, vomitting after eating and drinking. Pricking pain in the region of liver and under the right shoulder blade. Great constipation. Aggr. of pains by the least movement ; amel. by strong pressure, lying on the painful side These sympotoms develop after the abuse of calomel. Digestive troubles caused by cold and in summer.

Carduus Marianus. Intense heaviness of the head. Tongue white in the middle, the borders and the tips are red. Nausea, regurgitation, vomitting of green acid liquids. Alternate constipation and diarrhoea. Golden yellow stools and urines. Pain in the hepatic region and more particularly in the region of the right lobe of the liver. *Ceanothus*. Jaundice complicated with a big spleen which is hypertrophied.

Chamomilla. Tongue yellow, bitter taste eructations, nausea. Greenish stools. Stools and urines are hot and yellow.

Chelidonium. White coated pasty tongue, burning with the impression of the teeth, red borders and tip, thick saliva, loss of appetite. Dislike for food, nausea. Desire for hot drink. Alternate constipation and diarrhoea. Urine, bright yellow, sometimes with redish, viscous sediment. Pricking pains in the hepatic region. Spasmodic pain irradiating towards the back and right shoulder.

Chionanthus. Tongue covered with thick yellow coating, the month is dry which nothing ameliorates. Violent pain in the umbilical region ; sensation as if the intestines are tied, which constricts suddenly and relaxes slowly. Hypertrophied liver. Cement coloured stools. Black urine.

China. Tongue is yellowish, the lips dry. Bitter taste and eructations. Everything, even pure water tastes bitter. Marked swelling of the liver, causing troubles of respiration after meals. Putty like stools, frequent, foetid gas which does not ameliorate. Excoriating sensation in the right hyponchondria which is very sensitive to touch.

Hydrastis. The tongue is white, soft, having the imprints of teeth. Taste of copper or bitter taste in the mouth. The liver is small. discoloured stools, less abundant. Foetid urines.

Leptandra. Yellowish tongue. Bitter taste in the mouth. Sensation of fullness in the region of gall bladder. Pain in the hepatic region, irradiating to the backbone. Discoloured, or black as tar urine. Hemorrhoids.

Mercurius solubilis. Tongue soft, flabby with imprint of teeth. Salivation. Intense thirst, aggr. at night. Abundant sweats that does not relieve. Sweats may leave yellow patches on the linen. Diarrhoea, stools with teneasmus and straining. Turbid and red urine.

Myrica. Very marked jaundice with itching of the skin. Coated tongue. Thick, tenacious, nauseating saliva. Foetid breath. Bitter taste. Loss of appetite. Desire for acid things. Fullness in the region of liver. Urine less abundant, deep yellow. Colourless diarrhoeic stools.

Nux vomica. Tongue clear in the behind half, covered with yellowish white coating in the fore part. Sour taste. Nausea in the morning after meals. Epigastric region sensitive to touch. The liver is big with a sensation of heaviness and pricking pains. Characteristic constipation ; inefficacious need for stools.

Podophyllum. Wide, humid tongue. Putrid taste in the mouth. Thirst for large quantity of water. Vomitting of mucous. Sensation of distention of the abdomen, ameliorated lying down on the belly. Pain in the hepatic region, ameliorated by rubbing with the hand. Discoloured stools, hard difficult, with alternate diarrhoea. Haemorrhoids.

Taraxacum. Headache. Mapped tongue, white spots on some places, some parts seem excoriated. Big, indurated liver, which is acutely painful. Constipation.

CH. Noailles

GALL-STONE AND ITS COMPLICATIONS : VALUE OF HOMOEOPATHIC TREATMENT.

1. Dyspepsia at the Beginning.

We are going to review the field of Homoeopathic treatment of the different manifestations of gall-stone. It is only a few years ago this question was broached, not only because new remedies were proposed, but mainly because the French school could codify with precision and adapt in a sure manner in each well determined clinical case, some medicines used so long without any method. This should be for us a lesson of humility, because very often there was want of precision which hindered the homoeopath to obtain good results even using the more old remedies of the Materia Medica. It is a variable dyspepsia, with pain, sometimes *early* at the end of meals (Robinia type), sometimes *late* like that of an ulcer (*Nux vomica or Anacardium*), calmed after eating. But the characteristic of this pain is that the pain is due to indigestion of special foods : Fatty food, eggs, iced foods, chocolate etc. Sometimes even the *Aerophagia* reveals latent gall stone. When a radiographic plate is taken there is seen a vertical dislocation of the stomach (Faroy) and twisted pylora may be later on the seat of an ulcer. Sometimes the ulcer may be on the duodenum. For all these manifestations it is necessary to treat the patient in a strictly homoeopathic manner. In these cases one must remember the value of *Gratiloa, Nux vomica, Ignatia, Kali carbonicum* also of *Argentum nitricum* and also of the value of the ground remedies : *Thuya, Lycopodium, Graphitis* with *Nux vomica, Ignatia, Kali carbonicum* which are also remedies of temperament. Some times *Prandial Diarrhoea* is seen, which is a symptom of colitis as well as of the affection of gall bladder. This diarrhoea immediately after meals is seen in *Argantum Nitricum, China, Natrum Sulphuricum* (diarrhoea immediately after breakfast)

Alternate constipation and diarrhoea will indicate according to the case *Cheli Donium or Chionannus or Nux Vomica, Iris Versicolor, Jugluns Cinerea.*

2. Affections and Troubles of Duodenum.

The progress in radiography obtained since some years have shown the relation between *the Duodenum and the Gall Bladder* This is very important. There are two cases :

1. There may be *Duodeual Spasm* or even *Ulcer* formed after chronic dyspeptic troubles or more or less repeated dyspeptic troubles. In this case it is frequently seen that there is coexistence of functional troubles of the liver and of the bladder or there may already be vesicular lesions : *Choleaystitis*, with gall stone revealed or not in gall bladder.

In this cases, the ground remedy may be according to the temperament of the subject either *Thuja*, or *Natrum sulphuricum*, or *Lycopodium* (to be used prudently) and often *Phosphorus*, the most important remedy of temperament of Cholecystitis.

2. There may be some radiographic symptoms denoting the existence of a vesicular inflammation, *Cholecystitis and Pericholecystitis* , causing secondarily periduodenitis. There is then the *Adhesions.* If they are old, and organised they play the most important part in some painful phenomena. They should be treated by *Silicea* (groundremedy, high dilution 200 or M), followed by *Thiosinamine* (in high dilution according to Cahis of Barcelona) by *Calcarea Fluorica, Fluor ic Acid.*

What is interesting to note according to our personal opinion is that numerous patients from 40 to 60 years ot age who have a long and long series of dyspeptic and dudenal troubles with cholecystitis in the beginning or pericholecystitis and periduodenitis, have at the sametime a precancer state; their general condition becomes bad, they become emaciated, they have numerous new skin spmptoms : naevi, multiple warts etc. Often without X-ray the diagnosis is uncertain. And even when there certainly is not cancer one dose of *Micrococcin 200*, does good to them; they put on weight. One Kg. within 10 days. It seems that these patients have arrived at a cross road. Before them there are two divergent roads leading to the same point, the road to selerosis which leads to cirrhosis, and more or less advanced senility; the other road leads to cancer. The organism choses one or the other and according to our experience we may say that even in this stage we may help the patients not to fall in the one or the other danger. But if our remedies come late, one of the two roads are chosen and utilised and there remains no hope for complete cure.

3. Hepatic Colic.

It is not possible to deal with it here. Let us only mention here some very simple remedies specially from the vegetable kingdom, which will help us to get a rapid and favourable result.

A. The Pain Characteristics:

1. Dioscoria villosa and *Colocynthis* which oppose each other.

2. Bryonia, Belladonna, Atropinum sulph & Chamomilla, related to the two above.

B. Hepato-biliary insufficiency, concomittant or anterior to the crisis or which follows it will indicate.

3. *China, Berberis, Chelidonium, Chionanthus* in simple cases.

4. *Carduus marianus*, *Hydrastis*, *Arsenicum album* in more serious cases.

C. *The following constitutional remedies may also be used.*

5. *Calcarea carbonica*, *Nux vomica*, *Lycopodium*, *Phosphorus*, *Cholesterin.*

4. The cholecystitis and the stone of choledoch.

a. Limits of homoeopathic treatment and of surgery.

Before giving indications on the treatment of cholecystitis, let us precise first of all what are here the limits of actions of homoepathy and of surgery.

Chronic cholecystitis may lead towards sclero-atrophy. It is in this case specially the duodenum and even the pylora may be united together by adhesions, with the possibility of stenosis or pylora requiring surgical intervention. After clinical and radiogrphic examination of the stomach, intestines and and gall bladder, the physician will judge if the lesions are very chronic, inveterate. We homoeopaths will yield the place of homoeopathay to surgery.

Very rarely there will be hydrocholecystitis, the bladder increases in volume and distends behind a calculous obstruction. In some cases homoeopathy may cure and in some cases help of surgery should be taken.

Finally if the cholecystitis is suppurated, it should be operated except in cases treated early by homoeopathy where a resorption may be obtained. Our internal remedies, our compresses with M.T. of selected medicines will have an admirable effect, but if the time presses, if the general condition of the patient is grave and when a gangrenous cholecystitis is feared, it is necessary to take recourse to surgery immediately. Our therapeutic results obtained in most of the cases of simple cholecystitis is sufficiently good, but we must be prudent, impartial and believing in surgery.

b. Homoeopathy and Lithiasic Temperament.

But what is very important, is to recognise the lithiasic temperament, already described by Paracelsus and we should know how to treat it.

A—How strange is the diathesis that obliges numerous organisms to the necessity to form stones. The *Salivary Lithiasis*, tartars of the teeth, ranula (There are some persons who have too much tartar of the teeth, others have very little), renal lithiasis, biliary stones, patchiatic lithiasis ; intestinal or stercoral lithiasis, lithiasis of muscular and conjunctive tissues etc There is a *General Tendency to Calculus* ; that tendency seems often to have some nearest points and evolution with the *Tendency to Sclerosis*. It is due, some says to *Arthritism* ; to *Psora* say the disciples of Hahnemann. These different terms servel only to veiour ignorance, because still we do not know the why and how of the tendency to stone. It only appears that the persons who have it evolves in some cases more or less rapidly towards senility, sometimes in advance, as also seen to evolve in the same sense but still more rapidly, those who have the tendency to sclerosis or to fibrosis.

What are the habitual homoeopathic remedies of persons whose evolution is towards sclerosis ? *Thuya, Plumbum* and its salts, *Baryum* and its salts, *Aurum* and its salts, etc...and *Silica,* and *Iodium.*

For those who have the tendency to from stones, *Thuja Calcarea Carbonica, and* sometimes *Sulphur, Natrum Sulphuricum, Lycopodium.*

But bile stones are somewhat different from other stones. We know that chemically it is due to the deposit of Cholesterin. Cholesterin is a normal product of the blood. It is diminished in tuberculous patients and its use in gross doses will help cicatrisation in this disease. On the contrary it is increased in the blood of the plethorics who have the tendency to obesity or persons having hepato-biliary insufficiency. In persons suffering from hypertension an increase is also seen. In arteriosclerotic persons, persons suffering from Bright's disease and in some cases of pregnancy etc. What is the exact part played by cholesterin? Nothing is yet known. However it is known that it is antagonistic to lecithin and one finds almost always these two substances in the same case. By the side of hypercholesterinemia there is lipemia which is important to take into account and the phosphorated fat, lipoids in excess in the blood of some subjects having insufficient liver and the tendency to fabricate too much organic fat co-existing then with the increase of the percentage of cholesterin.

It seems then rational in these cases to try *Cholesterium* which seems to act better in high dilutions. It may be alter. nated with *Phosphorus* M, 200 or DM, every 8, 15, or 30 days. The effect is often remarkable. The patient no more fabricate calculus, and even if they exist, is not covered with a hard calcarious coating, We may cause diminution of their volume. Besides these cases, *often the percentage of cholesterin in the Blood remains the same or high* inspite of the general amelioration of the subject and also of the liver. It is therefore important to know the remedies that are indicated by lipemia which often leads to obesity and by hypercholesterinemia that may coexist with it or alone on its own account.

We have often mentioned these remedies. They are: *Phosphorous, Graphitis, Calcarea carbonica,* ***Natrum sulphuricum****, China, Cholesterinum* and possible also ***Lecithin*** in ponderable doses.

China is classic (Cartier). It prevents biliary lithiasis. ***Graphites, Calcarea carbonica. Natrum sulphuricum*** evolves towards obesity, with frequent lipemia and often cholesterinemia.

Phosphorus seems to me mervellously indicated in persons who have cholesterinemia and great thirst, who, like *Natrum Muriaticum*, and *Bryonia*, drink large quantity of cold water, drink much during meals, because cholesterin is avid of water.

Moreover *Phosphorous* acts on degenerescence, which may cause excess of cholesterin in the blood and the tissues (arteritis, cataract etc.)

This question has not yet been solved but it seems to play an important part and later on it will be necessary to know well the homoeopathic remedies indicated by laboratory findings, also by subjective symptoms or by objective symptoms that individualises the patient.

B—By the side of Cholesterin diathesis there is the infection factor. Some micro-organisms have been discovered in the nucleus of the stones. The infections therefore play a determinating part in person predisposed to lithiasis.

Besides, almost half of chronic cholecystics are not stone forming. Most of these cholecystitis which are not lithiasics are of intestinalorigin, and seen in patients who are constipated with right sided painful stasis. It is perhaps the infection of the liver: enterohepatic syndrom or there is entero-renal syndrom.

These patients are to be treated like cholecystitic lithiasic patients, predominantly by medicines of infection than by remedying the lithiasis. But often in these cases there is also high rates of cholesterin. There is therefore between the two cases very close relation and probably the same etiology: *Colibacillinum* may be used and *Enterococcin* as well.

By the side of these cases, the infection, insted of being colibacillary may be Eberth's bacillus. Cholecystitis of *Acute Typhoid Fever*, subacute or tending towards chronic stage. In these cases nosode *Eberihinum* may help.

But let there be infection or no infection the indicated remedies will generally be the same as those of lithiasic cholecystitis.

C—Hepato-biliary insufficiency.

In order that lithiasic cholecystitis is formed, there must be at the sametime hepato-biliary insufficiency with the formation of stone and infection.

The hepato-biliary insufficiency is more or less profound. But by interrogating the patient it is easy to find that it has developed in a latent manner during long period before the phase of confirmed cholecystitis.

This affection is of extreme frequency and develops for some general causes in relation to the modern life, the shocks of all sorts that it gives to our sensorial organs and to our overworked modern sympathetic system. Emotion, cares, different mental traumatisms and above all defective food, too rich in indigestible substances in our sedentary habits, cause soon hepato-biliary insufficiency. Hypercholesterinemia which predisposes to formation of gall stones is seen extraoridnarily frequent in all dyspeptics, plethorics, hereditary or acquired arthritics.

Infection causes later on by ascending passage or by descending passage, through blood particularly in case of Eberth's bacillus or paratyphic bacillus.

The evolution is variable. Very often cholecystitis exists alone but choledocitis may be associated; rarely there is angiocholitis with infection causing lesions up to the interior of the liver in and around the bile ducts. There are angiocholecystitis or chronic cholecystitis which may be subacute, evolving towards atrophic sclerosis of the bladder. Its evolution is slow, the temperature does not exceed 38 or 38.5. There are also some acute suppurated cholecystitis with puffiness of the hypochondria and vascular plastron. Finally there are over-acute or gangrenous forms which may suddenly show in the form of very grave genenralised peritonitis.

In case of these last two cases of acute or gangrenous cholecystitis immediate surgical recourse is to be taken. The homoeopathic remedies should yield its place to surgery or should be used as secondary treatment before and after the operation. But very often we will speak specially of it. What should be their therapeutics.

D—Search for a Rational Therapeutic of cholecystitis

In official medicine the dilemma is : should be operated or not ? When one should operate ? If the disease seems to be cured by itself in time and with much patience, regimen, rest and some therapeutic trials, one should think that it is fortunate to have such a result thanks to the chance of the patient and in such a case the doctor does not merit the result because the treatment is neither audacious nor complicated : Absolute rest, application of ice, diet which must be strict and which can cause rapid emaciation, prescriptions of some chemicals as medicine, that pretend to modify the intestinal content or disinfect it.

More rational is the use of cholagogs, when the content of the bile allows it. Because, in fact, it may be dangerous to mobilise the gall stone more or less voluminous by a brutal drive of the bile from liver to intestines. On this matter it is interesting to recall the trials that have been done to valorise and classify different eliminatory substance or substances forming bile. It is necessary to distinguish with Brugsch and Hörster, the property called *Cholagogs* and *Choleretics*. The cholagogs only eliminate the bile content in the extrahepatic bile duct and in the bladder. They are ***Magnesium Sulphuricum, Peptone, Olive Oil, Yellow of the Egg, Milk and even Simple Water*** and wine, finally Vichy water, water of Carlsbad and of Chatilguyon, But almost all the substances have value as preventives, only to check the cholecystitis. In the biliary infection, in the developed stage, their use is dangerous.

The choleretics directly increases the flow of the bile secretion not only in the liver, but within the tissues, on the surface of the interstitial lymphs and lacunary system. We may divide them in 5 groups (Charbol)

The Aromatic Group. Which corresponds to Atophan, Naphtolate and Oxynaphtolate of sodium or potassium, Biliary salts. Very active choleretics may be included in this group but not used in Homoeopathy.

The Fat Group. Oil of Haarlem, Oleic acids and Oleates, double product of oil and chloralose.

The Diastasic Group. Secretine, Histamin and possibly Insulin.

The Mineral Group. Sodium sulphate and Megnesium chloride, Calomel, the action is disputable and not well known. Nephtal, a new diuretic, is dangerous and rapidly toxic, having a mercury base.

The Vegetable Group. The bark of *alder*, root of *Eupatorium*, *Rizopoda*, flowers of *Rosemary* and of *Artichaks*, flowers and roots of *Chicorea*, *Aloe*, *Rhubarb*, *Cascara*, *Boldo*, *Mentha*, *Podophyllum*.

It is interesting to note here the scientific confirmation of our homoeopathic remedies such as *Eupatorium perf.*, *Taraxacum*, *Aloe*, *Rheum*, *Podophyllum*, in the vegetable group; *Natrum sulphuricum*, *Magnesia muriatica*, *Mercurius dulcis* (Calomel) in the mineral group. Compare also in the group of bile salts and in the oil group : *Calculi biliaris*, *Fel tauri*. As preventive the mineral waters may give good effect but they may be dangerous when the cholecystitis is confirmed.

Hepato-biliary organotheraphy should not be neglected. To homoeopaths also it may give good help as Barishac and

Martiny use it. Pancreatic opotheraphy should not be neglected according to the gravity of hepatic troubles and lesions of pancreas co-existing with cholecystitis.

In spite of these different medicines, the doctor has often no arm against an infection, increasing slowly and rapidly, of the gall bladder and specially if the fever rises, if the pain increases, if the contraction of the abdominal wall in the region of hypochondria persists, if the nausea auguments, if there is the danger of icterus or sub-icterus and finally if X-ray plates show one or many stones, surgical intervention is necessary but even then there is risk.

It is necessary to avoid the ablation of the gall bladder and try to cure medically and if such a result is not possible, the surgeon will try to do only cholecystostomy which is always preferable to cholecystectomy.

5. **Cholecystitis. Therapeutic plan.**

1. Biliary drainage. Cholagogs add choleretics.

Lower dilutions of *Solidago, Carduus Marianus Berberis Podophyllum, Taraxacum, Hydrastis.*

Decoctions of Taraxacum, Artichaks (leaves), Rosemary (leaves) wild Chicori (leaves), Boldo, Podophyllum.

Ponderable doses of ***Megnesia sulphurica, Magnesia muriatica.***

Haarlem oil (small doses at long intervals)

Olive oil, biliary salts

Mineral waters (with care)

1. Homoeopathic remedies properly called.

(*a*) **External Liver.** Compress imbibed with mother tinctures of ***Chelidonium, Berberis, Carduus marianus, Bryonia, Chionanthus, Colocynthis, Charmomilla, Dioscoria, China. Myrica.***

(*b*) **Internal Liver.** Pain. *Colocynthis Bryonia Dioscorea M agne sia Phosphorica.*

Infection : *Baptisia, Gelsemium, Eupatorium Perf, China, Arsenicum album, Echinaeea.*

The homoeopathic remedies indicated in the fever of cholecystitis are often the same as that of intermittent fevers because of the similarity of the temperature curve in both the cases, besides analogous clinical pictures.

Hepato-biliary insufficiency. (Use the ground remedies) *Ricinus communis, Cocculus, Nux vomica, Ipecac.*

The *Mercuries. Vipera, Anacardium, China, Chelidonium, Myrica, Chionanthus, Ptelia, Kali carbonicum, Juglans cinerea.*

Grcund remedics (or remedies of mobid temperament).

Phosphorus, very often

Arsenicum Album, Lachesis Lycopodium (with great care)

Natrum Sulphuricum, very often.

Rarely *Graphitis, Ignatia, Nux Vomica, Natrum Muriaticum, Sepia, Sulphur, Psorinum, Aurum Metallicum, Silicea Calcarea Carbonica.*

3. Isopathic Remedies and Nosodes.

Cholesterinum (200, 1000, 10,000)

Lecithin, Lutein (high dilutions)

Individual blood isopathy, stools or urines.

4. Organotheraphy. Three types of prescriptions :

—Substitutive organotheraphy. Ponderable doses.

—Excitant organotherapy. Lower tritutations or medium dilutions.

—Regulatory organotheraphy. High dilutions (100—10,000)

Extracts of liver, pancreas, ovaries, spleen, kidney, billiary calculus.

1. Drainage.

Two failures, about 8 years ago after habitual homoeopathic treatment led me to think about the question of drainage. I was not content to use different other remedies wich are not classic. I wanted at first to obtain a good drainage of the bile in my patients. Homoepathic organotherapy, particularly *Fel tauri* and *Bilis* in the 3rd and 6th dilutions appeared to me to act though in an inconstant manner. Among the organotherapic remedies the specialised products called *proxitasis* seemed to me to have interesting acton. But it was not sufficient. *Haarlem oil* seemed to me more satisfactory. This is a secret product of Holland of the 16th century, always used, contain different plants mixed with the essence of *Teribinthina* and *Sulphur*. I still use this compound. A good remedy of drainage is also *Magnesia sulphurica*; but it should be used in Allopathic doses as for example a tea spoonful every week. In this way colics in case of simple cholecystitis may be prevented.

In homoeopathy we know already as remedies of drainage *Soldago virga* and *Carduus marianus*. But these remedies are very little effective in confirmed cholecystitis. The theory of drainage formulated by Dr. A. Nebel of Lausanne which leads specially to the treatment of cases of bile and cholesterin retention, has some deductive value in therapeutics. Let us recall the action of *Carduus* on the left lobe of the liver, its constipation of frothy stools, difficult and hard, its tendency to jaundice, with dark pigmentation on the skin; its evolution towards cholecystitis and pigmentary cirrhosis or ascitis, its precancer state. We should know that the pain of Solidago is localised on the kidneys in the J. L. Petit's triangle or in the costo-vertebral angle, its rare urines which are thick, with thick and red-brick deposits; its suburral tongue and the bitter taste in the mouth. The decoction of Boldo may be used as a drainage remedy or one may use the plant in low dilutions but its action is inconstant and very slight. *Boldo* seems to act always in the case of bitter taste in the mouth.

Two homoeopathic remedies which are very important should be mentioned here. *Hydrastis* and *Taraxacum*. these remdies are to be given in 3 or 6.

Hydrastis. Acts very slowly. It is a remedy of mucous membranes, specially of those that covers the exterior conduits, with multiple folds. There is on the membranes in question, a thick, viscous and yellowish discharge. It is the 'thick bile' of ancient authors. Its habitual symptoms are bitter taste in the mouth, atonic dyspepsia with slow digestion and great weakness, possible jaundice. Pre-cancer stage.

Taraxacum. The Dandalion, is a very excellent remedy, very often underestimated, of torpid liver with stubborn constipation, bitter taste in the mouth, big and indurated liver, abdominal meteorism, mapped tongue white with red patches like islands. Salivation of hepatic origin. Night sweats. Fever with chill after meals. Pre-cancer stage

Podophyllum. Elective action on duodanum. May be used as a cholagog, if it is indicated by its vomitings of bile, clear yellowish and profuse diarrhoea early in the morning, accompanied by prolapsus of the anus. But in homoeopathic dilutions *Podophyllum* may often cause constipation. Therefore it is not considered as on ideal drainage remedy in the case of the stoppage of bile excretion.

Finally *Berberis* should not be neglected. It is a remedy of drainage type with its weakness, its hepatic insufficiency, its pains in the region of the left kidney, its thick urine, difficult and high colour

Really speaking all these remedies are not sufficient. It is necessary to act in a different way and on upper level.

—Act on the general condition and on the altered sympathetic system *i.e.* to say on the principal symptoms of the affection in question, pain, the defense symptoms, the fever, the infection.

—Finally act on the hepato-bilio-pancreatic insufficiency, the principal responsible factors of the cholecystitis.

2. Remedies Indicated by Pain and Fever.

I will not dwell on the remedies specially on *Colocynthis, Dioscoria Villosa, Chelidonium, and Bryonia.* They are well known.

Colocynthis. Colic of the liver after anger. Very violent spasmodic and crampoid pains, OBLIGING THE PATIENT TO BEND FORWARD WHICH AMELIORATES THE PAINS.

Diescorea Villosa. Is very often indicated in hepatic colic which FORCES THE PATIENT TO STRETCH AND BEND BACKWARDS FOR AMELIORATION. Irradiation of the pain from gall bladder to the chest, back and arms.

Chelidonium. CONSTANT PAIN BELOW ONE OR TWO CENTIMETRES OF THE LOWER ANGLES OF THE SHOULDER BLADE. Irradiation to the shoulders, specially to the right shoulder. Biliary complications of pregnancy. Possible jaundice. Big liver, painful. Discoloured stools with constipation.

Bryonia. PAIN AMELIORATED BY COMPLETE REST. Aggr. by movement which forces the patient to remain quiet. The liver is big and painful, Constipation of hard, voluminous, dry stools as if burnt.

By Fever.

Different remedies have been used in cholecystitis. Such as : *Baptisia*. In the case of Eberth's bacillus and of para-typhoid, very grave with septicemia, delirium; dry yellowish tongue "Parrot tongue", hebetude, foetidity of breath and of the excretions. BED SEEMS VERY HARD.

Eupatorium Perfoliatum. INTENSE PAIN OF THE BONES OF THE EXTREMITIES AS IF THEY ARE BROCKEN. H.gh fever. Bitter taste in the mouth. Painful liver. Great thirst. Hiccough. MARKED PERIODICITY.

Gelsemium. Great shivering, specially aggravated at 10 in the morning. FEVER WITHOUT THIRST. Adynamia with nausea. Intermittent fever.

I must admit that I have very little experience about the classic remedies of fever as regards biliary infection except *Gelsemium* of which I had an important case which proved its value. On the contrary the remedies indicated by pain *Bryonia, Colocynth, Chelidonium, Dioscorea* are very important to consider, because, as I have noted, they may have a rapid calming effect on an infected and painful gall-bladder.

But above all, in these cases, one should know how to use these remedies externally, in compress on the liver. This method is neglected by the homoeopaths and they are worng. Here is how one proceeds. The M.T. should be used because even the lower dilutions do not act, or act less. The patient should apply on the region of the liver a big compress of double flanel, humid and soaked with water, then pressed. The water according to the case and the modalities of the remedy may be used, cold, hot or tepid. On this compress sprinkle some drops of (5 to 10) of M.T. of two or three medicines. Naturally a mixing of a number of tinctures should be avoided, because the action will be less and it will not be possible to know the tincture of which the action is optimum. In our practice the mother tinctures that we apply are those of *Berberis, Cheldonium Bryonia, Chinanthus, Myrica and China*, and sometimes *Disoarea Cococynthis, Eupatorium.* The sedative action is rapid ; the pain ameliorates and above all the contraction and the perivesicular plastron becomes soft and finally dis appears. Thus one may avoid dangerous abcess and peritonitis. In acute cases the compress may be left on the liver and made humid every three or four hours with re-impregnation with the tinctures. In chronic cases where the patient is not bed-ridden, and who may move here and there during the day, the compress may be kept on the liver at night. The sedative action is undeniable and much more superior to using ice, cold or hot compresses.

3. The Remedies of Hepatic Insufficiency.

It remains now the study of the most important remedies of cholecystitis ; those which may attack the cause itself, hepato-biliary or hepato-bilio-pancreatic difficiency. These remedies may not only be preventive but also curative which are very important to take into account, being given that habitually this infection comes slowly, after a long phase of dyspeptic and hepatic troubles, and after successive appearences.

I will not study in detail the symptoms of all these remedies, which will be long and fastidious. I will speak a few words only on those that are well known, but I will speak in detail about those that are less known and proposed since recently though they are very important to know.

Are known by all :

China. Abdominal meteorism, big liver, big spleen, jaundice. Liquid non-digested stools. Weakness. Sensitiveness to touch, to contact, to air-current.

Chelidonium. Already described.

Myrica. Bitter and nauseating taste, anorexia, painful liver, discoloured stools, intestinal gas, charged urine, insomnia.

Chionanthus. Jaundice, big and painful liver, constipation, soft pasty and discoloured stools. Anorexia, big spleen *Periodic Hepatic Pains.*

The Mercuries. Specially *Mercurium dulcis.*, Nausea, vomiting, diarrdoea with incessant desire for stools and the sensation of having no end. Salivation, foetid breath. Thirst with humid mouth. Flabby yellow tongue, having imprint of of the teeth. Tendency to cirrhosis of liver. Possible jaundice.

Juglans Cineria. Choleolithiasis. Sensitive liver, gastric distension. Occipital headache.

Ptelia. *Cannot lie down on the left side.* Eructations, vomiting, nausea, vomiting and weakness. Abdominal meteorism.

Kali Carbonicum. Frequent nausea, better by lying down. Flatulence. Weakness. Sweats. Lumber pains. Possible jaundice. *Pricking as if by Needles on the Region of Liver* ("Stitches")

Nux Vomica. Nausea in the morning, after meals. Vomiting which is difficult. Epigastric sensitiveness to pressure. Big, sensitive liver ; constipation with inefficacious desire. Sedentarism. Abuse of stimulants.

These are classical remedies. Only *Vipera* and *Ricinus communis* are not generally well known. Both are of great value, specially the second one. These remedies are very much used by *Dr. William Bas,* but priority goes to *Gallivardin.*

Vipera is a valuable remedy. Boerick is proud of this remedy. Big painful liver. Jaundice and fever ; pain irradiating to shoulder, to right hips. Dry, brown tongue. Veins are swollen on legs. Pains of the legs or of the liver with *Bursting Sensation. Cannot keep the Legs Hanging.*

Ricinus communis is a mervellous remedy and cures immediately the nausea of hepatic origin or biliary nausea. Anorexia, nausea, *Vomiting.* Dry mouth. Diarrhoea possible with colic or very often without pains. Fever, emaciation and somnolence.

I give *Ricinus* in fixed times according to the time of nausea as stated by the patient as for example, in the morning after waking up or very often at four in the evening in order to check the aggravation from 5 to 8 p.m. in relation to *Lycopodium*, the ground remedy. *Ricinus* is also a good complementary of *Phosphorus* in hepatic insufficiency and *cholecystitis*.

It remains for us to study the ground remedies, remedies of temperament of chosecystitis, remedies that are to be used at long invervals, rarely repeated and in high dilutions.

In these cases, though they are rare, *Calcarea Carbonica*, *Aurum metallicum*, *Sulphur*, *Sepia*, *Graphitis* may be used according to the symptoms presented by the patient.

More often symptoms of *Natrum Sulyhuricum*, *Lachesis and Arsenicum* are seen.

Natrum sulphuricum is a well known remedy for elimination of bile containing in the gall-bladder. It suits to hydrogenoid patients having big or torpid liver. Diarrhoea is more frequent than constipation, coming specially in the morning immediately after break fast.

Lachesis often acts deeply on the liver. It antidotes *Vipera*. So it is related to it. It suits to women in time of Lachesis menopause, cholecystitis after stoppage of menses. Amelioration after the return of menses.

Arsenicum Album. It may be frequently indicated as a ground remedy (it may be given in medium or in lower dilutions) of worn out patient, suffering since long-time from *cholecystitis*, restless and prostrated at the sametime. Nightly aggravation from one a.m. or from midnight to 3 a.m.

But the two great ground remedies of cholecystitis that are the most frequently indicated are *Lycopodium* and *Phosphorus*.

Lycopodium and Phosphorus. Both used in deficient liver, but in a different way. *Lycopodium* or vegetable *sulphur* recalls to us by the outline of its pores, the form of hepatic lobula. *Lycopodium* is also easily combustible. It contains besides *Sulphur* and is related more to *Sulphur* than to *Phosphorus* medically. It is much less violent than the latter and should not act deeply like the other on the hepatic cells. The mentality of *Lycopodium* is also very different from *Phosphorus. Lycopodium* is quarrelsome, often agggresive, angry, extremely irritable, violent in his words and in his letters. *Phosphorus* is at first exalted, over-active, then prostrated. *Lycopodium* acts on the bile excretion and elimination of toxins that come out of the muscular activity. *Lycopodium* is bilious par excellence. "It is the remedy of bitter". *Phosphorus* on the contrary is the remedy of sugar troubles, it destroys the glycogene. It acts on the blood and on the walls of the vessels. *Lycopodium* is not indicated in both these cases. *Phosphorus* has deep action and is used in still more grave cases and often, we may say, that a patient who was formerly a patient of *Lycopodium* has come to be the patient of *Phosphorus. Phosphorus* is the most important remedy of fatty degeneration, *Lycopodium* never.

But the value of *Phosphorus* in high dilutions is not yet known in acute and specially in chronic *cholecystitis.*

In almost all the cases of *cholecystitis* that I have treated since 8 years, I have arrived at complete success by *Phosphorus* M, when drainage was assured by *Berberis, China, Bayonia, Ricinus communis.* The last one is a marvellous remedy of nausea of hepatic origin.

Lycopodium should be used with great precaution because it is often dangerous in persons suffering from cholecystitis who do not drain themselves.

It is necessary to begin with 6 or 12 to rise later on to 30, 200 and M rarely repeated.

Phosphorous on the contrary is not dangerous in this case (It is dangerous only in laryngeal tuberculosis). It acts mervelously in high dilutions, preferably M. I use it alternately with *Cholesterium M*.

By the side of *Phosphorus*, it is necessary to use in cholecystitis three new remedies on which I must insist. *Cholesterinum*, *Lutein*, *Lecithin*.

Cholesterinum is well studied in the last editions of Boerick. I do not agree with the opinion of the author abow the dilutions. He recommends the 3x. All the lower dilutions and triturations have given me no good result. Even the 30th hardly acts. *Cholesterin* is active only in high dilutions 200 or M. What is curious is that when it is aternated with *Phosphorus* M, it ameliorates *cholecystitis* but does not bring down the cholesterin of the blood.

China is the classical remedy of hypercholesterinemia. Really speaking *China*, *Phosphorus* and *Cholesterin* act on the bad result of excess of *Cholesterin*. An alimentary regimen is necessary at the same time to lower down the cholesterin content of the blood. *Lecithin* is the physiological opposit of *Cholesterin*. It contains phosphorus which cholesterin does not. *Lecithin* is a phosphorated fat contained in the brain and in the yellow of egg. I have used it successfully on the indications of *Phosphorus* in 200 and M. It is perhaps the first trial, because this use is not indicated in the books. It is used olny in convalescence, in tubercular patients, in insomnia, in neurasthania and for nurses who have not sufficient milk. One of its good indication is the presence of large quantity of phosphate in the urine.

Lutein. It was first used by our friend Martiny. It is used in medium dilutions 30 or high 200 or M, in hypercholesterinemia and *cholecystitis* of menopause. It acts marvellously on this type of women.

—

A SIMPLE EXAMPLE OF HOMOEOPATHIC PRESCRIPTION IN CHRONIC CHOLECYSTITIS

It requires too much time to know homoeopathy well and we do not wish to discourage those who come to homoeopathy by our study which is surely very long. Let those who want to appreciate homoeopathy, try it in order to be the impartial witness of the results that they may obtain.

It is only for this reason we are going to give here a very simple example of homoeopathic prescription, which we do often and on in our daily practice, when we have to treat a chronic cholecystitis. The remedies that we are going to enumerate are for the treatment of the starting of the disease. They are simple to prescribe, easy to use by the patient. Our homoeopath friends will reproach us for being too much schematic by giving this example which is contrary to the law of Hahnemann.

In fact the homoeopathic treatment should always be adapted to the patient and not to the diseases and we must avoid routinism. But we may say that seven times out of ten it will be advantageous to begin thus the treatment of a subject suffering from chronic *cholecystitis*. Prescribe then these remedies for three months even if these remedies are less indicated by the symptoms described above.

Prescribe.

Phosphorus 200, 2 doses, the first dose at the begining of the treatment, the 2nd dose ten days after the 1st (the best remedy that may act on gall bladder)

Bryonia 30, two granules every day in the mornning after waking up in the morning.

Ricinus communis 6, 2 granules at 4 p.m.

China 30, 2 granules every evening while going to bed.

These remedies are also given according to their time modalities. *Bryonia* seems often to act in this case after meals at night, time of amelioration. *Ricinus communis* given after noon relieves nausea and dyspeptic troubles, *i.e.* to say a bit before the habitual stage of aggravation of hepatics, those that are suited to *Lycopodium* and *Chelidonium* etc. aggr. towards 5 in the evening, finally *China,* complimentary of *Phosphorus* seems to act better at the end of the day.

Berberis 6, 5 drops in a small quantity of water before noon meals (hepato-biliary drainage)

Compress in the evening and keep it the whole night sprinkled with 5 to 10 drops of *Bryonia* M.T., and *Chelidonim* M.T.

But routinism should be avoided and one should know how to modify this prescription by replacing the remedies not indicated by the patient with those that are indicated. One will already obtain a sedation of pains, the diminution of temperature, and amelioration of hepato-biliary symptoms, the region of the gall bladder will be softer by palpation, it will be less tense and less painful.

In graver cases the treatment should be done in different manner at the sametime by drainage and canalisation of the toxins.

By the side of good results obtained in this way what can a unicist do by his single remedy given in high dilution as a ground remedy ? We have tried this method formerly, but such a practice is deceiving and sometimes even dangerous. The necessity of drainage is absolute, still more so in the treatment of hepato-biliary affection. This is a glaring confirmation of the value of the theory of drainage and canalisation of Dr. A. Nebel.

THERAPEUTIC PLAN OF HOMOEOPATHIC TREATMENT OF CIRRHOSIS AND DIFFERENT HEPATOMEGALIS.

Cirrhosis.

We must know that even in grave cases of degeneration whether it is the question of cirrhosis of Laenac, different diffused or fatty forms, cirrhosis of Hanot, hypertrophic, syphilitic, pigmentary etc...that in spite of the gravity of such diseases as cirrhosis, in spite of the clinical picture which is so accentuated, clinical evolution which seems irremediable, and the great difference that exists in the anatomy between a healthy and a cirrhotic liver, Homoeopathy may obtain here some really extraordinary results. The patient may live for a longtime even if he is an old alcoholic one; the puncture for ascitis becomes rarely necessary. I have often seen the ascitis to disappear not to appear again (on condition that it is still less developed and puncture is not done). It is absolutely necessary to avoid puncture that precipitates the patient toward the formation of new hydropsy and hasten his death, and it is remarkable to be able to obtain such results in patients gravely and irremediably attacked. I remember the case of a patient whose condition was very grave, who had the picture of arythmia, anasarca, ascitis, and hypertrophic cirrhosis. The quantity of urine passed during 34 hours was only 200 to 300 CM^3. Every time I gave him *Phosphorus* 200 at first and M afterwards the quantity of urine increased to 1.800 or 2,000 cm^3 the next day of the dose. Then it gradually came down at the end of a week. The action of the remedy stopped. The quantity of urine reached to 200 to 300 cm^3. I prescribed *Phosphorus* again. I continued to treat the patient for two years and the ascitis disappeared as well as the oedema of the legs. No puncture was necessary. This case proves the extraordinary effect of *Phosphorus.*

We will give simply a classification of the remedies of cirrhosis.

Classification of the Remedies of Cirrhosis.

We will distinguish here ·

a. Ground remedies : *Phosphorus, Lycopodium, Lachesis, Arsenicum album.*

b. Remedies indicated by anatomy, pathology as reproducing experimentally some cirrhotic liver, or indicated by anatomic disorders :

Sclerosis. *Aurum Muriaticum Natronatrum, Aurum Metallicum, Plumbum Metallicum, Silica, Iodum, Arsenicum Album.*

Kali Iodatum, Mercurium and its Salts (*Merc. iod. rubr.* and *Merc. dulcis*) in case of syphilis (besides *Aurum, Aurum mur. natronatrum,* and *Plumbum*).

Graphitis Taraxacum Fluoric Acidum indicated by INDURATION OF THE LIVER.

Fatty Degeneration. *Kali bichromicum, Phlorizin Vanadium, Picric acid* (besides *Phosphorus*).

Pigmentary degeneration. Argentum nitricum.

Pre-cancer and Cancerous Evolution. *Cholesterinum* (besides *Carduus marianus, Taraxacum, Conium, Hydrastis*)

c. Remedies Indicated by Etiology.

Ethyl-Alcohal the remedy of Cahis may be tried in the cirrhosis of Laenac.

T.R. and other *Tuberculins* for the tuberculosis.

Luesinum for syphilis.

Let us note here that the remedies indicated by pathological anatomy are almost all minerals, while clinical remedies indicated by symptoms of the liver are all vegetables. Now we are going to enumerate them.

Let us arrange them into groups :

Remedies of the First Importance. *Carduus Marianus, China, Seneceo, Chelidonium Hydrastis, Mercurius, Dulcies, Nasturium Ag, Nux Vomica, Ricinus Communis.*

Remedies of the 2nd Importance. *Abis canadensis, Calcarea arsenica, Cascara, Cocculus indicus, Natrum chloride, Nitric acid, Natrum muriaticum and Podophyllvm, Quassio.*

Remedies of Ascitis. (besides Carduus marianus, China, Seneiceo) *Appocynum cannabinum, Digitalis, Acetic acid, Prunus spinesa.*

Organotherapic and Drainage Remedies).

Hepatic organotherapy.

Fel tauri, Fel porci.

Magnesia sulphurica (avoid overworking the liver).

Oil of Haarlem etc...

Hepatomegalis.

This is also a very complex question which requires long study. Let us give only some useful indications.

A. How to Adapt Homoeopathic Therapeutic to Passive Congestion of Liver.

1. In my opinion there are three important remedies which are to be used in high dilutions, 30, 200, M, DM.

Sulphur. Arrteial hypertension (big liver). Benignant cases. Good myocardia. Tendency to cutaneous eruptions.

Natrum Sulphuricum. Hydrogenoid constitution, oliguria, diminution of blood viscosity.

Phosphorus. *Grave cases. Weakss of the right heart* Bile retention. Evolution towards cardiac cif hosis. Oliguria, sub-icterus, ascitis. Weakness of the myocardia.

Tendency to fatty degeneration of the heart and liver. Cardiac tuberculosis of children (*Phosphorus* and *Silicea Silicea* in the case of symphysis of the myocardia.

Rarely, *Sepia*, *Lachesis*, *Pulsatilla* or other remedies of the ground in high dilution.

Homoeopathic remedies of the first importance indicated by the symptoms.

Digitalis. Before all other remedies. It should be used in all possible dilutions. *It has the Superiority to act not only Homoepathically but also Physiologically.*

Grave, urgent cases. Digitalis 5 drops, or maceration of Digitalis leaves.

In other cases Digitalis 1x, 3x, or 1 then 6, 30, 200. In some cases give only the 200 which will depend on the patient. Good remedy of accordeon liver. Asystole or Hyposystole. Sub-icterus. Slow, irregular pulse, trigeminal pulse. Oliguria and tendency to oedema or to ascitis

China. Tendency to oedema and ascitis. Tendency to *cholesterinemia*; the *cholesterin* is avid of water, whence the dehydration of the organism which is however swollen and more or less oedematous. Peri-visceral oedema. Debility, because these retained organic liquids are physiologically useless and lost at least momentarily for the organism. Bitter taste in the mouth. Tendency to icterus and urobilinuria.

Podophylum. Painful liver. pain amel. by friction on the right hypochondria. Constipation of hard stools and discoloured stools, or often foetid yellow, diarrhoea, in the amorning. The liver at first big, becomes later on small. Elective action on the duodenum.

Apocynum Canabinum. Tendency to oedema and to ascitis. Weakness of the *Right Heart*, specially of the triscupid valves. Turbid urine. Acute alcoholism.

Kali Carbonicum. Tendency to oedema and ascitis. Chill, weakness, *pain in the back. Sudden fleeting*, stinging pain. *Lancinating Pain.*

These remedies are studied in detail on the chapters of icterus and cirrhosis.

Use also external homoeopathic treatment : A few drops of the two indicated remedies, to be imbibed in a humid flanel, placed on the liver for several hours during the day or the whole night.

B. Active Congestion of the Liver.

It is translated in a reaction of the hepatic parenchyma, against intoxications and infections.

It is seen in the first stage, before cirrhosis in *Alcoholism* Malaria is also a frequent cause. *China* type.

It may be due to over eating. *Sulphur* and *Nux vomica* types.

It may be due to intestinal stasis, chronic constipation : *Magnesia muriatica* type.

It may be due to a real infection of the liver (typhoid, pneumonia)

The liver is painful *by Palpation.*

The Principal Remedies of Active Congestion of the Liver.

We are enumerating them only as they are already studied.

Beginning. *Aconite, Bryonia, Chamomilla.*

Developped. *Mercurius solubilis, Mercurius dulcis, Cholidonium, Podophyllum, Chionanthus, China, Nux vomica, Berberis, Myrica, Iris versicolor.*

Grave Cases. *Vipera, Arsenicum album, Phosphorus, Lachesis.*

Tendency to Abcess or Suppuration. He*par sulphur.*

It is necessary to use with care, the ground remedies : *Phosphorus, Sulphur, Lachesis, Sepia, Natrum Sulphuricum.* These remedies are already studied.

Chronic Cases or Tendency to Chronicity. *Ammonium muriaticum, Cholesterinum, Kali iodatum, Kali muriaticum, Kali bichromicum, Iodium, Hydrastis* and the remedies already indicated for the beginning and for the developped stages of acute congestion.

In Alcoholics. *Ammonium muriaticum, Arsenicum album, Absinthium, Fluoric acid, Leptandra* and as remdy of temperament *Sulphur, Lachesis* and *Phosphorus.*

The Portal Hypertension and Hemorrhoids. *Aloe, Aesculus hippocastum, Leptaedra* and as remedies of temperament *Sulphur, Sepia, Nux vomica.*

When Pain is Aggravated Lying on the Left Side. *Ptelia, Bryonia, Natrum sulphuricum.*

pain Aggravated Lying on the Right side, *Magnesia muriatica, Mercurius, Chelidonium, Dioscoria, Kali carbonicum.*

Pain Ameliorated by Friction. *Podophyllum.*

Pain and Congestion of the Left Lobe. *Carduus marianus.*

Concomittent Splenomegalis. *Ceanothus.*

Pain with the sensation of imminent diarrhoea, mapped tongue, large vesicul ar eruptions. ***Rananculus sceleratus.***

For active congestion use external application as indicated at the end of passive congestion of the liver.

C. **Tuberculosis of the Liver.** Tuberculosis may be associated with alcoholism to create cirrhosis.

There is also fatty hypertrophic eirrhosis of Autinel and Galarin.

There is moreover cardiac-tubercular cirrhosis already mentioned in relation to the passive congestion of the liver.

Moreover fatty degeneration is frequent in advanced pulmonary tuberculosis.

Finally there is amyloidosis after tuberculosis with cavity, or bone tuberculosis suppurating for a long time, big liver, big spleen, diarrhoea, renal amyloidosis.

Treatment. The best remedy is *Phosphorus.* But it is dangerous in cases of evolution of pulmonary tubrculosis.

Other remedies of fatty degeneration : *Kali bichromicum, Phlorizin , Vanadium, Picric acid, Aurum muriaticum.*

Naturally you will use the diluted *Tuberculins* according to the case : *Spengler, Marmoreck, Bacillinum, Denys, Aviary, K. T., R. T.* The most indicated are *Bacillinum* and R.T.

D. Hepatic Syphilis.

Secondary Syphilis. Sometimes catarrhal icterus.

Tertiary Syphilis. Sclero-gumman lesions : big hard liver, lignous, tied up, sometimes atropho-hypertrophic, according to the lobes. Sclerous bands. Sometimes of pseudo tumoral form. Spontaneous pains caused by perihepatitis. Splenomegalis. Frequent albuminuria. Sometimes ascitis. Frequent bile retention. Evolution towards sclerosis. Irregular fever. Sometimes hypertrophic cirrhosis with chronic icterus.

Treatment : *Syphilinum, Aurum metallicum, Aurum muriaticum, Plumbum metallicum, Kali iod., Mercurius solubilis, Mercurius dulcis.* These are the classical remedies.

Don' t forget if indicated: *Phosphorus, Sulphur, Lycopedium* (with care).

The treatment of kystes (hydratic) and abcess of the liver, clearly surgical, goes beyond the limit of our study.

Specific classical treatment which is still sure, cyanide of Hg, preferably intra-venous (avoid mineral salts, because dangerous).

□ □ □